KV-213-022

INSTANT NURSING ASSESSMENT:

$\mathscr{R}$espiratory

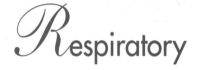

▽   ▽   ▽   ▽   ▽   ▽   ▽

Mary L. Wilby, RN, C, MSN, OCN
Pain Management Coordinator/Clinical Nurse Specialist
Temple University Cancer Center
Philadelphia, Pennsylvania

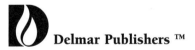

Delmar Publishers ™

I(T)P™ An International Thomson Publishing Company
Albany • Bonn • Boston • Cincinnati • Detroit • London • Madrid
Melbourne • Mexico City • New York • Pacific Grove • Paris • San Francisco
Singapore • Tokyo • Toronto • Washington

$\mathcal{S}$TAFF

Team Leader:
DIANE McOSCAR

Sponsoring Editors:
PATRICIA CASEY
BILL BURGOWER

Developed for Delmar Publishers by:
JENNINGS & KEEFE Media Development, Corte Madera, CA

Concept, Editorial, and Design Management:
THE WILLIAMS COMPANY, LTD., Collegeville, PA

Project Coordinator:
KATHLEEN LUCZAK

Editorial Administrator:
GABRIEL DAVIS

Production Editor:
BARBARA HODGSON

Manuscript written by:
TERRI A. GREENBERG

Text Design:
KM DESIGN GROUP

For information, address:
Delmar Publishers
3 Columbia Circle
Box 15015
Albany, NY 12212-5015

International Thomson Publishing Europe
Berkshire House 168-173
High Holborn
London, WC1V7AA
England

Thomas Nelson Australia
102 Dodds Street
South Melbourne, 3205
Victoria, Australia

Nelson Canada
1120 Birchmount Road
Scarborough, Ontario
Canada M1K 5G4

International Thomson Editores
Campos Eliseos 385, Piso 7
Col Polanco
11560 Mexico D F Mexico

International Thomson Publishing GmbH
Königswinterer Strasse 418
53227 Bonn
Germany

International Thomson Publishing Asia
221 Henderson Road
#05-10 Henderson Building
Singapore 0315

International Thomson Publishing Japan
Hirakawacho Kyowa Building, 3F
2-2-1 Hirakawacho
Chiyoda-ku, Tokyo 102
Japan

COPYRIGHT© 1996 BY DELMAR PUBLISHERS

The trademark ITP is used under license.

Printed in the United States of America

Published simultaneously in Canada by Nelson Canada, a division of The Thomson Corporation.

1 2 3 4 5 6 7 8 9 10 XXX 00 99 98 97 96 95

Library of Congress Cataloging-in-Publication Data
Wilby, Mary L., 1957-
    Instant nursing assessment: respiratory/Mary L. Wilby.
        p. cm. — (Instant nursing assessment)
    Includes bibliographical references and index.
    ISBN 0-8273-7099-7
        1. Respiratory organs—diseases—nursing. 2. Nursing assessment. I. Title. II. Series.
        [DNLM: 1. Respiratory Tract Diseases—nursing. 2. Nursing Assessment—methods. WY 163 W666i 1995]
    RC735.5.W53 1995
    610.73'692—dc20
    DNLM/DLC
    for Library of Congress   95-371
                                                               CIP

$\mathcal{T}$ITLES IN THIS SERIES:

Suzanne K. Marnocha, RN, MSN, CCRN
Assistant Professor, College of Nursing
University of Wisconsin
Oshkosh, Wisconsin

Linda Moody, RN, FAAN, Ph.D.
Professor, Director of Research and Chair,
Gerontology Nursing
College of Nursing
University of South Florida
Tampa, Florida

Patricia A. O'Neill, RN, CCRN, MSN
Instructor, DeAnza College School of Nursing
Cupertino, California

Virgil Parsons, RN, DNSc, Ph.D.
Professor, School of Nursing
San Jose State University
San Jose, California

Elaine Rooney, MSN
Assistant Professor of Nursing, Nursing Department
University of Pittsburgh
Bradford, Pennsylvania

Barbara Shafner, RN, Ph.D.
Associate Professor, Department of Nursing
Otterbein College
Westerville, Ohio

Elaine Souder, RN, Ph.D.
Associate Professor, College of Nursing
University of Arkansas for Medical Sciences
Little Rock, Arkansas

Mary Tittle, RN, Ph.D.
Associate Professor, College of Nursing
University of South Florida
Tampa, Florida

Peggy L. Wros, RN, Ph.D.
Assistant Professor of Nursing
Linfield College School of Nursing
Portland, Oregon

$\mathcal{C}$ONTENTS

NOTICE TO THE READER

The publisher, editors, advisors, and reviewers do not warrant or guarantee any of the products described herein nor have they performed any independent analysis in connection with any of the product information contained herein. The publisher, editors, advisors, and reviewers do not assume, and each expressly disclaims, any obligation to obtain and include information other than that provided to them by the manufacturer.

The reader is expressly warned to consider and adopt all safety precautions that might be indicated by the activities described herein and to avoid all potential hazards. By following the instructions contained herein, the reader willingly assumes all risks in connection with such instructions.

The publisher, editors, advisors, and reviewers make no representations or warranties of any kind, including but not limited to the warranties of fitness for particular purpose or merchantability, nor are any such representations implied with respect to the material set forth herein, and the publisher, editors, advisors, and reviewers take no responsibility with respect to such material. The publisher, editors, advisors, and reviewers shall not be liable for any special, consequential, or exemplary damages resulting, in whole or in part, from readers' use of, or reliance upon, this material.

A conscientious effort has been made to ensure that the drug information and recommended dosages in this book are accurate and in accord with accepted standards at the time of publication. However, pharmacology is a rapidly changing science, so readers are advised, before administering any drug, to check the package insert provided by the manufacturer for the recommended dose, for contraindications for administration, and for added warnings and precautions. This recommendation is especially important for new, infrequently used, or highly toxic drugs.

CPR standards are subject to frequent change due to ongoing research. The American Heart Association can verify changing CPR standards when applicable. Recommended Schedules for Immunization are also subject to frequent change. The American Academy of Pediatrics, Committee on Infectious Diseases can verify changing recommendations.

FOREWORD

As quality and cost-effectiveness continue to drive rapid change within the health care system, you must respond quickly and surely—whether you are a student, a novice, or an expert. This *Instant Assessment Series*—and its companion *Nursing Interventions Series*—will help you do that by providing a great deal of nursing information in short, easy-to-read columns, charts, and boxes. This convenient presentation will support you as you practice your science and art and apply the nursing process. I hope you'll come to look on these books as providing "an experienced nurse in your pocket."

The *Instant Assessment Series* offers immediate, relevant clinical information on the most important aspects of patient assessment. The *Nursing Interventions Series* is a handy source for appropriate step-by-step nursing actions to ensure quality care and meet the fast-paced challenges of today's nursing profession. Because more nurses will be working in out-patient settings as we move into the 21st century, these series include helpful information about ambulatory patients.

These books contain several helpful special features, including nurse alerts to warn you quickly about critical assessment findings, nursing diagnoses charts that include interventions and rationales along with collaborative management to help you work with your health care colleagues, patient teaching tips, and the latest nursing research findings.

Each title in the *Instant Assessment Series* begins with a review of general health assessment tools and techniques and then expands to cover a different body system, such as cardiovascular, or a special group of patients, such as pediatric or geriatric. This focused approach allows each book to provide extensive information—but in a quick reference format—to help you grow and excel in your specialty.

Both medical and nursing diagnoses are included to help you adapt to emerging critical pathways, care mapping, and decision trees. All these new guidelines help decrease length of stay and increase quality of care—all current health care imperatives.

I'm confident that each small but powerful volume will prove indispensable in your nursing practice. Each book is formatted to help you quickly connect your assessment findings with the patient's pathophysiology—a cognitive connection that will further help you plan nursing interventions, both independent and collaborative, to care for your patients skillfully and completely. With the help and guidance provided by the books in this series, you will be able to thrive—and survive—in these changing times.

— Helene K. Nawrocki, RN, MSN, CNA
Executive Vice President
The Center for Nursing Excellence
Newtown, Pennsylvania
Adjunct Faculty, La Salle University
Philadelphia, Pennsylvania

SECTION I. GENERAL HEALTH ASSESSMENT REVIEW

Chapter 1. Health History

▽ ▽ ▽ ▽ ▽ ▽ ▽

*I*NTRODUCTION

SEE TEXT PAGES

When taking a health history, collect critical subjective data about the patient. In addition to collecting clues about existing or possible health problems, you are also drawing a road map for future patient interactions. To make this map as useful as possible, gather information about the patient's physical condition and symptoms and explore the patient's psychological, cultural, and psychosocial environment as it pertains to his or her health issues.

*B*EGINNING CONSIDERATIONS

Collecting vital information about the patient can be a daunting task. Patients are often nervous and apprehensive. They may also feel awkward or embarrassed about sharing their problems and concerns, particularly if they've never seen you before. You may even feel some anxiety about the prospective interview.

You can do several things to ease the situation:
• Create a comfortable physical environment.
• Learn interviewing techniques that will put the patient at ease.

*T*HE EXTERNAL ENVIRONMENT

The external environment is the place where you meet with the patient to collect the health history.

Do the following to help the patient feel at ease:
• Conduct the interview in a quiet, private area.
• Set the thermostat at a comfortable level.
• Make sure the lighting is adequate.
• Avoid interruptions.
• Remove objects that might upset or distract the patient.
• Position yourself and the patient as equals by:
  - Sitting in comfortable chairs at eye level. Standing implies that you are more powerful.
  - Not interviewing the patient from behind a desk or table.

- Maintain an appropriate distance between you and the patient. Be sensitive to cultural differences and the need for personal space.

Communicating with Your Patient

Successful communication requires good interpersonal skills that place the patient at ease. To do so, use the techniques suggested by the acronym DEAR:
- Demonstrate acceptance
- Empathize openly
- Affirm
- Recognize

The best way to show a patient that you accept what he or she is saying is to listen. People know that you are listening when you make comments like "I see what you are saying" or simply, "I understand." When you nod your head yes and make eye contact, you also show that you are attentive and accepting of what you hear. Acceptance is not the same as believing the patient's statements are right or wrong.

Empathy is the uniquely human ability to put yourself in someone else's shoes, to show that you can relate to his or her feelings. You show empathy when you say such things as "That must have made you sad/frightened/happy/relieved."

When you affirm and recognize, you are putting acceptance and empathy to work. Affirmation is the act of acknowledging what the patient is telling you.

Recognition is listening well and attentively, thus showing the patient by what you say and how you say it that you hear him or her. It can be as simple as nodding yes or saying "Please continue."

Some patients will come to you with as many concerns about the treatment process and environment as about their health. Reassure them that all communication is confidential and that you cannot legally reveal anything beyond the confines of the health care team without the patient's consent.

*E*NSURING A SUCCESSFUL INTERVIEW

Sometimes patients are so apprehensive or have had such negative health care experiences that they are hostile. To best handle such a patient, follow these guidelines:

• Remain calm.
• Never argue with the patient.
• Affirm and recognize his or her feelings using simple sentences.
• Reschedule the interview if the patient's hostility persists.
• If you feel physically intimidated by the patient, call for assistance.

A second factor that can skew the results of your interview is a cultural or ethnic difference between you and the patient. Differences between cultures can be subtle. For example, in the United States, most people consider it rude not to make eye contact. Culturally, the absence of eye contact suggests disinterest or dishonesty. In many other cultures, it is considered extremely rude to make eye contact with elders or authority figures, or eye contact is not made between unrelated members of the opposite sex.

While it is important to be sensitive to cultural differences, try not to go to the other extreme and resort to stereotyping. Each of us is a unique individual regardless of our culture. No one perfectly embodies all the characteristics of a culture.

Sometimes we use the term "ethnic group" to refer to a group that shares a common culture. At other times we use the same term to refer to a group that shares a common biological origin. On still other occasions we use the term to refer to a group that shares a common national origin. Beware of making judgments about a patient's behavior based on biological ethnicity. Skin color is not a good predictor of cultural affiliation. People who are "American" come in all sizes, shapes, and colors.

Pay attention to how culture and individual character affect the patient's lifestyle, fears and hopes about his or her health, and feelings about treatment. This can be an exciting journey for both of you.

*T*HE INTERVIEW: YOUR ROLE

The interview involves two persons—you and the patient—and is really the sum of what both of you bring to it. You, however, are the authority figure, and most patients will expect you to set the tone and direction of the interview. Your goal is to help the patient become a willing participant in his or her own care—to actively assist in discovering solutions to problems he or she may experience. The more you know about successful interviewing techniques, the more likely you are to be at ease with the patient. Remember: These techniques are general guidelines. You are the best judge of what is most effective in any given situation.

Like a college essay, the interview can be broken into three parts: the introduction, the main body (the interview), and the conclusion (parting with the patient).

*T*HE INTRODUCTION

The introductory phase of the interview sets the tone for the rest of the assessment. It's also where you begin to build a rapport with the patient.

- Always start the interview by introducing yourself and giving the patient some background on your place in the organization. It may help to shake hands. Always ask the patient how he or she likes to be addressed.
- Take a little time to get to know the patient by talking informally before you begin the interview process.

NURSE ALERT:
Make sure the patient speaks fluent English. If not, you may want to postpone the interview until you can obtain an interpreter.

- Explain how long the interview will take.
- Describe the interview process and ask the patient for questions.
- If you need to take notes to remember information, tell the patient you will be doing so in order to listen more attentively.

*T*HE INTERVIEW

The main body of the interview is where you collect the information you need for the patient's treatment and care. Provide a road map. Begin the interview process by asking general questions. Ask the patient why he or she came in for today's visit. During the interview, help the patient by asking questions such as "Is there anything else you're worried about?"

Repeat important points the patient makes. You can make a comment such as "You just said that your pain occurs early in the morning. Let's explore that for a second."

Another way to draw the road map is to interpret what the patient has said and done. You could say, "It sounds like whenever you are short of breath, something has happened to make you anxious." Clarify the patient's statement as much as possible.

In other situations, the patient may have trouble verbalizing his or her concerns. In this case, a response like "It seems to me that you are concerned about..." shows that you will do whatever is necessary to help the patient communicate more clearly.

Finally, you can help the patient be clear by summarizing major points with statements such as "So far, we've talked about...I think we are ready to go on to talk about...."

Give the patient time to think about what he or she needs to say. This shows that you respect the patient's thought process. Use silence to focus on the patient's nonverbal behavior.

Be an observer. Be aware of the patient's unspoken behavior. When appropriate, use these observations for clarification and to heighten the patient's awareness. Simple observations such as "It appears that that must have been a painful experience" often open new avenues for exploration and discovery.

Affirm the patient's role in the interview as a participant. For example, ask the patient to offer strategies for dealing with his or her health care issues.

Sometimes patients may make statements or have expectations that are unrealistic. Respond by pointing out the obvious—"You told me your side doesn't bother you, but you wince every time I touch it." Or you might say, "You'll feel much better after treatment, but you won't be able to go back to long-distance running."

It is very important that the patient remain grounded. Comments such as "You look worried," "You seem tense," and "You sound more relaxed" affirm the patient's feelings.

You can empower patients to be willing participants in the interview process by openly sharing whatever information and facts you have about their health care and the decisions involved in it. Clearly explain patient care and how the health care system works.

Avoiding Pitfalls

Just as there are good techniques for interviewing, there are techniques to avoid because they increase tension and reduce communication between you and the patient.

- Justification. When you ask patients how or why something happened, you are implying that they need to explain or defend their behavior. You can also make a patient feel you expect an explanation when you ask leading questions. A leading question always implies that there is a single "right" answer. For example, "You don't eat a lot of fried foods, do you?" is likely to get a no from even the most dedicated french-fry eater.
- Too persistent. There is an old saying about not beating a dead horse that applies to interviews. If you don't get the desired information after a couple of tries, move on.
- The wrong tone. Be careful to gear your discussion to the patient's ability to understand it. On the one hand, don't overwhelm the patient with technical terms and medical jargon. On the other hand, don't talk down to the patient.

Pay attention to how the patient prefers to be addressed. For example, an older woman may find it patronizing and rude if you address her by her first name.

If you are talking about death, use statements such as "he died," not "he's gone to his reward." Pay attention to such euphemisms when used by the patient. They are a way to avoid real feelings, and we most often resort to them when talking about subjects that make us feel anxious or frightened.

Be personable but not personal. If you begin to share your own experiences or provide advice, you are likely to make the patient feel like a nonparticipant in the health care process.

The patient who asks for advice is demonstrating respect and trust. You can repay that with responses such as "Even if I were in the exact same situation as you, I might not want to do the same thing. What do you think is best for you?"

While touch can be comforting to a patient, too much of it can feel inappropriate. Likewise, be aware of becoming too impersonal. When you assume the posture of an authority figure, you create distance between you and the patient. To say, "I'm the nurse and I know best," even when a patient is clearly doing something destructive like smoking, implies that the patient is inferior to you.

Another way to be too impersonal is to use impersonal language. It is the difference between "That wasn't very clear" and "I don't understand." The first statement removes you from the equation. Also, consider the following:

• Losing touch with reality. Making statements such as "It will all be OK," "Don't worry, you'll be fine," or "Life goes on" may make you feel better, but they don't make the patient feel better. Rather, the patient is likely to feel that you don't care about the impact of his or her illness or that you cannot be trusted to tell the truth.

• Interrupting. If you interrupt the patient or change the subject, you are likely to make the patient feel that you are impatient. The same is true of drawing conclusions too quickly. When you draw all the conclusions, the patient is likely to withhold information or tell you what he or she thinks you want to hear.

• Inappropriate emotion. Inappropriate responses to what the patient says include the following:
  - Don't overly praise the response. If, for example, our french-fry eater said no to your leading question about fried foods and you responded with "That's fantastic. It's great that you're so disciplined," you're not likely to find out what his diet and exercise patterns really are.
  - Don't show disapproval or anger.
  - Don't take the patient too literally. If a patient says he is not afraid of needles but pulls his arm away, shuts his eyes, and grits his teeth, he is clearly apprehensive about injections. It's important that you base your response as much on what the patient does as what the patient says.

𝒫ARTING WITH THE PATIENT

How you close the interview is as important as how you open and conduct it. Ask the patient if he or she has any other questions or comments and how he or she feels about the treatment decisions. Summarize the information collected in the interview and any decisions that have been made about future treatment. Make sure you and the patient understand this in the same way.

𝒩ONVERBAL CUES

Not all communication is spoken. In fact, the majority of communication is nonverbal. You can learn to send non-verbal messages to your patient that emphasize the qualities of DEAR discussed earlier in this chapter.

- Appearance. Be appropriately professional. Avoid dressing in a way that makes the patient uncomfortable.
- Posture. Be relaxed. Keep your arms uncrossed to convey openness. Direct your body toward your patient. Don't slouch.
- Gestures. Occasionally, you can use your hands to encourage conversation. Touch the patient's arm for comfort. Never point at the patient, clench your fist, or drum your fingers. Avoid looking at your watch. Never touch the patient in a way that he or she may find inappropriate.
- Facial expression. Try to look actively interested. Smile and show concern when appropriate. Avoid yawning, which expresses boredom. Try not to frown, grimace, or chew on your lip or cheek. Maintain appropriate eye contact.
- Speech. Keep your voice moderate. Raise it only if the patient has trouble hearing. Watch your tone of voice with patients who speak English as a second language. We all have a tendency to yell when trying to make ourselves understood. Make sure you are not speaking too quickly or too slowly.

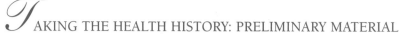

AKING THE HEALTH HISTORY: PRELIMINARY MATERIAL
Having laid out the structure of the interview, it is now
time to get down to specifics. Each institution has its own
form. Be complete in filling out the form specific to your
institution. The table that follows lists initial information
you should obtain from your patient.

NURSE ALERT:
If the patient is feeling ill, begin by collecting the relevant
information about his or her illness. Collect other information afterward or reschedule the patient. Don't tax the
patient's energy with the interview.

HEALTH HISTORY CHECKLIST

AREA TO COVER	SPECIFIC QUESTIONS
Biographical information	Use the form your institution provides.
Allergies	Are you allergic to any: • medications (include reaction) • foods (include reaction) • environmental agents (include reaction)
Medication	What medications (including dosages) do you take on a regular basis? Include both prescription and over-the-counter medications.
Childhood illnesses	Have you had measles, mumps, rubella, chicken pox, pertussis, strep throat, rheumatic fever, scarlet fever, poliomyelitis?
Accidents or injuries	Describe and include dates of any accidents or injuries you've had.
Chronic illnesses	Do you have diabetes, hypertension, heart disease, sickle cell anemia, cancer, AIDS, seizure disorder?

HEALTH HISTORY CHECKLIST (CONTINUED)

AREA TO COVER	SPECIFIC QUESTIONS
Hospitalizations	Describe, including dates and diagnoses, any hospitalizations.
Surgical procedures	Describe, with dates and diagnoses, any operations.
Obstetric	How many times have you been pregnant? How many full-term pregnancies have you had? Have you had any abortions?
Immunizations	Did you receive the complete battery of childhood immunizations? What is the date of your most recent tetanus shot, hepatitis B vaccine, tuberculin skin test, flu shot?
Last examination	When were your most recent physical, dental, and eye examinations; hearing test; ECG; and chest X-ray performed?

PHYSIOLOGICAL ASSESSMENT: GENERAL

> The following table lists general physiological questions to ask the patient. If the patient is not feeling well, go on to the table titled "Current Complaint." If possible, also cover the family history information listed in the "Family Environment" table.

AREA TO COVER	SPECIFIC QUESTIONS
Present health status	Have you had any recent weight gain or loss? Do you know the cause? Do you experience any of the following? • fatigue, weakness, or malaise • difficulty in carrying out daily activities • fever or chills • sweats or night sweats • frequent colds or other infections Are you able to exercise?
Skin	Do you have a history of any of the following: • eczema, psoriasis, or hives • changes in pigment • changes in any moles • overly dry skin • overly moist skin • excessive bruising • pruritus • rashes • lesions • reaction to heat or cold • itching • sun exposure and amount Describe the location of any growths, moles, tumors, warts, or other skin abnormalities.

PHYSIOLOGICAL ASSESSMENT: GENERAL *(CONTINUED)*

AREA TO COVER	SPECIFIC QUESTIONS
Hair	Describe any recent hair loss, change in hair texture, or change in hair characteristics. How often do you shampoo your hair? Is your hair color-treated or permed? How often do you have this done?
Nails	Have you experienced any of the following: • changes in nail color • changes in nail texture • occurrences of nail splitting, cracking, or breaking • changes in nail shape
Head and neck	Have you experienced any of the following: • frequent or severe headaches • dizziness • pain or stiffness • a head injury • abnormal range of motion • surgery • enlarged glands • vertigo • lumps, bumps, or scars
Eyes	Have you been troubled by any of the following? • eye infections or trauma • eye pain • redness or swelling • change in vision

PHYSIOLOGICAL ASSESSMENT: GENERAL (*CONTINUED*)

AREA TO COVER	SPECIFIC QUESTIONS
Eyes (*continued*)	Have you been troubled by any of the following? • eye infections or trauma • eye pain • redness or swelling • change in vision • spots or other disturbances of the visual field • twitching or other sensations • strabisimus or amblyopia • itching, tearing, or discharge • double vision • glaucoma • cataracts • blurred vision, blind spots, or decreased visual acuity Do you wear glasses? Do you have a history of retinal detachment? When did you last have a glaucoma test and what was the result?
Ears	Have you experienced any of the following? • ear infections or earaches (include dates and frequency) • hearing loss • tinnitus (ringing or crackling) • exposure to environmental noise • discharge from the ear—color, frequency, and amount • vertigo • unusual sensitivity to noise • sensation of fullness in the ears When did you last have an ear examination? What was the result? What impact does your hearing loss have on your daily activities? How do you clean your ears?

PHYSIOLOGICAL ASSESSMENT: GENERAL *(CONTINUED)*

AREA TO COVER	SPECIFIC QUESTIONS
Nose	Do you have a history of the following? • nosebleeds • nasal obstruction • frequent sneezing episodes • nasal drainage—color, frequency, and amount • trauma or fracture to the nose or sinuses • sinus infection (include treatment received) • allergies • postnasal drip • pain over sinuses • change in the sense of smell • difficulty breathing through nose
Mouth and throat	Do you have a history of the following? • oral herpes infections • mouth pain • difficulty chewing or swallowing • lesions in mouth or on tongue • tonsillectomy • altered taste • sore throat (include dates and frequency) • bleeding gums • toothache • hoarseness or change in voice • dysphagia When did you last have a dental examination? What were the results? What is your daily dental care regiment? Do you wear dentures or any other type of dental appliance?

PHYSIOLOGICAL ASSESSMENT: GENERAL *(CONTINUED)*

AREA TO COVER	SPECIFIC QUESTIONS
Respiratory system	Do you have a history of any of the following? • asthma • bronchitis • tuberculosis • shortness of breath-if so, preceded by how much and what type of activity • coughing up blood • noisy breathing • pollution or toxin exposure • emphysema • pneumonia • chronic cough • chest pain with breathing • wheezing • smoking How much sputum do you cough up per day? What color is it?
Cardiovascular system	Have you experienced any of the following? • chest pain • heart murmur • need to be upright to breathe, especially at night • swelling in arms or legs • hair loss on legs • anemia • cramping pain in the legs and feet • leg ulcers • palpitations • color changes in fingers or toes • coronary artery disease • varicose veins • thrombophlebitis • coldness, numbness, or tingling in the fingers or toes Do you have hypertension, high cholesterol levels, or a family history of heart failure? Do you smoke? How many packs per day?

PHYSIOLOGICAL ASSESSMENT: GENERAL *(CONTINUED)*

AREA TO COVER	SPECIFIC QUESTIONS
Cardiovascular system *(continued)*	Do you sit or stand for long periods? Do you cross your knees when sitting? Do you use support hose?
Urinary tract	Do you have a history of any of the following? • painful urination • difficulty or hesitancy in starting urine flow • urgency • flank pain • cloudy urine • incontinence • frequent urination at night • pain in suprapubic region • changes in urine • decreased or excessive urine output • kidney stones • blood in the urine • pain in groin • bladder, kidney, or urinary tract infections • low back pain • prostate gland infection or enlargement
Gastrointestinal system	Have you experienced any of the following? • appetite changes • dysphagia • indigestion or pain associated with eating (obtain symptoms) • vomiting blood • ulcers • gallbladder disease • colitis • constipation • black stools • hemorrhoids • food intolerance • heartburn

PHYSIOLOGICAL ASSESSMENT: GENERAL *(CONTINUED)*

AREA TO COVER	SPECIFIC QUESTIONS
Gastrointestinal system *(continued)*	• burning sensation in stomach or esophagus • other abdominal pain • chronic or acute nausea and vomiting • abdominal swelling • liver disease • appendicitis • flatulence • diarrhea • rectal bleeding • fistula How often do you have a bowel movement? Have there been any changes in the characteristics of your stool? Do you use any digestive aids or laxatives? What kind and how often? **THE ELDERLY:** For patients over age 50, obtain the date and results of last Hemoccult test.
Male reproductive system	Do you have a history of any of the following? • penile or testicular pain • penile discharge • hernia • sexually transmitted disease • sores or lesions • penile lumps • prostate gland problems • infertility How often do you perform testicular self-examination? Are you satisfied with your sexual performance? Do you practice safe sex?

PHYSIOLOGICAL ASSESSMENT: GENERAL *(CONTINUED)*

AREA TO COVER	SPECIFIC QUESTIONS
Female reproductive system	Do you have a history of any of the following? • excessive menstrual bleeding • painful intercourse • vaginal itching • bleeding between periods • missed periods • infertility • painful menstruation Provide the following information: • menstrual history, including age of onset, duration, amount of flow, any menopausal signs or symptoms, age at onset of menopause, any postmenopausal bleeding • satisfaction with sexual performance • date of last period • understanding of sexually transmitted disease prevention, including AIDS • number of pregnancies, miscarriages, abortions, stillbirths • date and results of last Pap test • contraceptive practices • vaginal discharge and characteristics **THE ELDERLY:** Ask elderly patients if they have experienced vaginal dryness or other problems.

PHYSIOLOGICAL ASSESSMENT: GENERAL *(CONTINUED)*

AREA TO COVER	SPECIFIC QUESTIONS
Breasts	Have you experienced any of the following? • nipple changes • nipple discharge—color, frequency, odor, amount • rash • breast pain, tenderness, or swelling Have you ever breast-fed? When was your last breast examination? What were the results? Do you perform breast self-examination? When did you last have a mammogram? What were the results? (for women over age 40)
Neurologic system	Do you have a history of any of the following? • seizure disorder, stroke, fainting, or blackouts • weakness, tic, tremor, or paralysis • numbness or tingling • memory disorder, recent or past • speech or language dysfunction • nervousness • mood change • mental health dysfunction • disorientation • hallucinations • depression Do any of these problems affect your day-to-day activities?
Musculoskeletal system	Do you have a history of any of the following? • arthritis or gout • joint or spine deformity • noise accompanying joint motion • fractures • joint pain, stiffness, redness, or swelling (include location, any migration, time of day, and duration)

PHYSIOLOGICAL ASSESSMENT: GENERAL *(CONTINUED)*

AREA TO COVER	SPECIFIC QUESTIONS
Musculoskeletal system *(continued)*	• other pain (include location and any migration) • problems with gait • limitations in motion • muscle pain, cramps, or weakness • chronic back pain or disk disease • problems running, walking, or participating in sports Do any of these problems affect your day-to-day activities?
Immune system	Do you have a history of any of the following? • anemia • low platelet count • blood transfusions (include any reactions) • chronic sinusitis • conjunctivitis • unexplained swollen glands • bleeding tendencies, particularly of skin or mucous membranes • HIV exposure • excessive bruising • fatigue • allergies, hives, itching • frequent sneezing • exposure to radiation or toxic agents • frequent, unexplained infections Do any of these problems affect your day-to-day activities?

PHYSIOLOGICAL ASSESSMENT: GENERAL *(CONTINUED)*

AREA TO COVER	SPECIFIC QUESTIONS
Endocrine system	Do you have a history of any of the following? • excessive urine output • unexplained weakness • changes in hair distribution • hormone therapy • nervousness • inability to tolerate heat or cold • endocrine disease, for example, thyroid or adrenal gland problems, diabetes • increased food intake • excessive thirst • goiter • excessive sweating • tremors • unexplained changes in height or weight • changes in skin pigmentation or texture (In addition discuss the relationship between the patient's weight and appetite.)

PHYSIOLOGICAL ASSESSMENT: CURRENT COMPLAINT

The following table provides a guide to collecting data about the patient's current complaint. Always begin by having the patient describe, in his or her own words, the reason for today's visit.

AREA TO COVER	SPECIFIC QUESTIONS
Time frame	When did the discomfort or alteration in pain start? Is it intermittent or constant? Is it worse at certain times of day?
Location	Where is the pain located? (Have the patient show you.)
Quality	Describe the pain. Is it sharp or dull? How severe is it?

PHYSIOLOGICAL ASSESSMENT: CURRENT COMPLAINT (*CONTINUED*)

AREA TO COVER	SPECIFIC QUESTIONS
Environment	Are there specific places or activities that seem to trigger the pain? Does anything relieve the pain? Make it worse?
Perception	What do you think your symptoms mean?

ASSESSING FUNCTIONAL STATUS

In addition to collecting specific physiological data, you need to assess the patient's ability to function on a day-to-day basis. The table below provides guidelines for such an assessment.

AREA TO COVER	SPECIFIC QUESTIONS
Daily activities	• What do you do during an average day? Does your complaint interfere with this? If so, in what way? • Do you exercise? If so, what type of exercise do you perform and how often do you exercise? Does your complaint interfere with exercise? If so, in what way? • Do you use street drugs? If so, how often? How has this affected you in terms of work and family?
Sleep and rest	• How long do you sleep? Need to sleep? • Do you have any difficulty falling asleep or staying asleep? • Do you wake during the night to urinate? How often? • Do you feel rested each morning? • Do you feel tired during the day?

ASSESSING FUNCTIONAL STATUS (*CONTINUED*)

AREA TO COVER	SPECIFIC QUESTIONS
Nutrition	• What have you had to eat or drink in the past 24 hours? Is this a typical daily diet? • Who buys and prepares food in your family? • Is the family income sufficient for the family food budget? • Does the family eat together? • How much caffeine from coffee, tea, or soda do you drink in a day? • When did you last have an alcoholic beverage? What do you drink and how much? Have you ever had a drinking problem?
Stress factors	• Do you live alone? • Do you know your neighbors? • Is the neighborhood safe or high in crime events? • Can you keep the temperature in the house comfortably warm or cool? • Are safety factors at work or in the home a stress factor? • What stressors would you list as present in your life now and in the past year? • Has anything about this stress level changed? • Have you ever tried anything to relieve stress? How well did it work?

FAMILY AND SOCIAL ASSESSMENT

It's particularly important to explore the patient's family history and relationships. The health history provides important clues about the patient's state of health and about how family relationships affect treatment and care.

FAMILY ENVIRONMENT

> The following table provides questions you can ask the patient that will help build a picture of his or her family environment. However, these questions imply a nuclear family structure. If the patient comes from a single-parent, gay, or extended family, you will need to modify them accordingly.

AREA TO COVER	SPECIFIC QUESTIONS
Mortality data on blood relatives	What is the age and health of your living blood relatives (parents, grandparents, siblings)? At what age did other relatives die and what was the cause of death?
Family history	Is there any family history of diabetes, heart disease, high blood pressure, stroke, blood disorders, cancer, sickle cell anemia, arthritis, allergies, obesity, alcoholism, mental illness, seizure disorder, kidney disease, tuberculosis?
Spouse and children	What are the ages and health condition of your spouse and children?
Patient's position within the family (The purpose of these questions is to find out how tasks are divided within families with children and to explore family health promotion, factorsthat are very important to patient care.)	• Are you happy with the set of tasks that you and your partner do as spouses and as parents? • Are there differences of opinion about child-rearing? How do you work out any differences? • Do you work outside the home? How does the family support you in your work? • Who is the primary caretaker of the children or older adults in the family? Are you happy with this arrangement? • Who makes doctor appointments, keeps track of medication schedules, and so on?

FAMILY ENVIRONMENT *(CONTINUED)*

AREA TO COVER	SPECIFIC QUESTIONS
Patient's position within the family *(continued)*	• Are you comfortable with how your children are maturing? Are they learning skills like hygiene, good eating habits, appropriate sleep and rest patterns? • Can family members share or switch tasks? Do they have the skills to do so? • Do you and your children have the same values? • If you are the caretaker, how will your family adjust to your illness?
Patient's views of the economics of the family	• Is your family income adequate to supply its basic needs? • Who makes the money decisions in your family?
Patient's support (These questions will help you understand your patient's social skills, the extent to which the patient has access to a support system, and if the patient is likely to feel isolated and depressed.)	• Do you belong to any clubs or organizations outside the family? What do you enjoy about them? • Whom do you ask for help and advice outside your immediate family? • How do you interact with your co-workers? • What do you like to do with your friends? How often do you get to do it? • Are you happy with your friendships? • What do you know about community agencies that can help you while you are ill and recovering?

FAMILY ENVIRONMENT *(CONTINUED)*

AREA TO COVER	SPECIFIC QUESTIONS
Patient's perception of family	• What is the place of family in your life? • Does your extended family include close friends? • Does anyone who is not a member of your immediate family live in your home? • How do family members interact? • Do they see each other in a positive light? • How do family members react to each other's needs and wants? Are positive and negative feelings expressed openly? • How does the family handle conflicts?

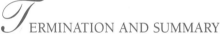

ERMINATION AND SUMMARY

End your interaction with the patient with the following:
- Summarize important information collected during the interview as well as the results of the interview and any conclusions you have drawn from it.
- If there are issues about health education—for example, contraception—either schedule a health education session or provide the patient with the information.
- Make any necessary referrals. Help the patient set up the appointment.
- Summarize decisions you and the patient have made about future care.
- Explain the physical part of the health assessment in detail.
- Ask the patient if he or she has any other concerns or questions.

DOCUMENTING THE INTERVIEW

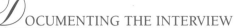

How you document what you have learned from the patient is as important as how you conduct the interview. Other health care professionals will use the patient's record as a basis for future care and treatment. It is important that you allow yourself adequate time to reflect on what the patient has told you and the most effective way to communicate that to other professionals in writing. Observe the following guidelines:

• Use the correct form.
• Use an ink pen, not a pencil.
• Write the patient's name and identification number on each page.
• Make sure the date and time appear with each entry.
• Use standard abbreviations that everyone will understand.
• Wherever possible, use the patient's description of symptoms.
• Wherever possible, be specific, not vague. Do not generalize.
• Do not leave anything blank. If something is not applicable, write "N/A" in that space.
• Do not backdate an entry.
• Never write on a previous entry.
• Never document for anyone but yourself.

*C*hapter 2. Physical Assessment Skills

▽ ▽ ▽ ▽ ▽ ▽ ▽

*I*NTRODUCTION

SEE TEXT PAGES

In the first chapter we explored techniques for the subjective portion of the health history. In this chapter we explore techniques for the objective portion—the physical assessment. This portion of the assessment will either confirm or bring into question the conclusions you and the patient drew during the subjective assessment. It can generate new avenues of exploration.

*T*OOLS OF THE TRADE

You yourself provide the most important equipment used in the assessment—your eyes, ears, nose, and fingers. What you see, hear, smell, and touch is critical. You will supplement those tools with special equipment. At a minimum, you will require a measuring tape, penlight or flashlight, thermometer, and visual acuity chart. You will also need additional basic equipment to complete the assessment. (See chart below.)

ASSESSMENT TOOLS

TOOL	USE
Wooden tongue depressor	Assess the patient's gag reflex and obtain a view of the pharynx.
Safety pins	Test the patient's sensation of dull and sharp pain.
Cotton balls	Test the patient's sensation of fine touch.
Test tubes of hot and cold water	Test the patient's ability to distinguish temperature.
Common substances, like coffee or vinegar	Test the patient's ability to smell and taste.

ASSESSMENT TOOLS (CONTINUED)

TOOL	USE
Disposable latex gloves	When handling body fluids (taking blood, rectal, and vaginal assessment)
Water-soluble lubricant	Assess rectum and vagina.

SPECIALIZED ASSESSMENT TOOLS

You may find that you need more specialized equipment to complete your assessment. Such equipment may include one or all of the following: reflex hammer, skin calipers, vaginal speculum, goniometer, transilluminator, ophthalmoscope, nasoscope, otoscope, and tuning fork. These tools require additional training to use correctly.

TOOL	DESCRIPTION	USES
Ophthalmoscope	Light source with a system of lenses and mirrors	Examine the internal eye structure: • Use the large aperture for most patients. • If the patient has small pupils, use the small aperture. • Use the target aperture to localize and measure fundal lesions. • Use the slit beam to measure lesion elevation and the anterior eye. • Use the green filter to determine specific fundal details.

NURSE ALERT:
You can adjust the intensity of light, but it's best to begin at the lowest level to avoid causing discomfort to the patient.

SPECIALIZED ASSESSMENT TOOLS (CONTINUED)

TOOL	DESCRIPTION	USES
Otoscope	Light source similar to the ophthalmo-scope.	Examine the external auditory canal and tympanic membrane.
Nasoscope	Three types: •Nasal speculum •A speculum for the nostrils that you attach to an ophthalmoscope •Handle like an ophthalmoscope, with short, slim head with light source	Examine the nasal interior. **!** **NURSE ALERT:** If you are not skilled in the use of the nasoscope, do not use it. You can cause the patient discom-fort.
Tuning fork	Shaped like a fork. Tines are designed to vibrate.	Check hearing and sensation.

DRAPING AND POSITIONING TECHNIQUES

Before you begin the actual assessment, you need to understand how to position and drape the patient. The correct technique varies, depending on the body area you are assessing. This table provides a quick description of draping and positioning techniques.

BODY AREA	POSITION	DRAPING
Head, neck, and thorax	Patient sits on edge of examination table.	None
Neurologic	In some cases, patient needs to to stand or sit.	None

DRAPING AND POSITIONING TECHNIQUES (CONTINUED)

BODY AREA	POSITION	DRAPING
Musculoskeletal	In some cases, patient needs to stand or sit.	None
Breast exam	Phase one: Seated Phase two: Supine, with pillow or towel under the shoulder on the side you are examining; have patient place arm on that side above her head.	None
Abdomen	Supine	Towel over female patient's breasts; for both sexes, sheet draped over lower half of body; do not pull the sheet below the pubic area
Cardiovascular	Supine	Sheet draped over torso and legs
	Sitting	Sheet draped over areas not being auscultated
Rectal (male)	Bent over the examination table or lying on left side	None
Rectal or reproductive (female)	Lithotomy position	Sheet draped over chest and knees and between legs

Assessment Techniques

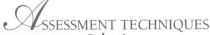

Palpation

You will use palpation, or different kinds of touch, throughout the assessment. Generally, palpation will follow inspection.

It is particularly important to palpate the abdominal or urinary tract systems at the end of the assessment. Otherwise, you may cause the patient unnecessary discomfort and distort findings.

During the assessment, you are likely to use four types of palpation. Light palpation requires a gentle touch with just the fingertips. Do not indent the skin more than 3/4 in (2 cm). If you push too hard, you will dull the sensation in your fingertips.

Deep palpation is more aggressive and usually involves both hands. Depress the skin 1.5 in (4 cm). Place the opposite hand on top of the palpating hand, using it as a control and guide. Use this technique to locate and examine organs such as the kidney and spleen or to anchor an organ like the uterus with one hand while examining it with the other. A variation on this technique involves using one hand to depress the skin and then removing it quickly. If the patient complains of increased pain as you release pressure, you have discovered an area of rebound tenderness.

NURSE ALERT:

If you use this variation during an examination of the abdomen and the patient feels rebound tenderness, consider the possibility that the patient may have peritonitis.

Light ballottement is a variation on light palpation. Using your fingertips, move from area to area, depressing the skin lightly, but quickly. Be sure to maintain contact with the patient so that you can identify tissue rebound.

Deep ballottement is a variation on deep palpation. Using your fingertips, move from area to area, depressing the skin deeply, but quickly. Be sure to maintain contact with the patient's skin.

Percussion

With percussion, you use your fingertips or hands to tap areas of the patient's body. Tapping can be used to make sounds, to find tender areas, or to judge your patient's reflexes. When used for sound, percussion requires specialized training and the ability to distinguish between slight differences in the sounds produced. Move from areas that make clear sounds to dull areas.

There are three percussion techniques: indirect, direct, and blunt.
- Indirect percussion involves both hands. Place the second finger of your left hand if right-handed or your right hand if left-handed against the appropriate body area—for example, the abdomen. Use the middle finger of your other hand to sharply and quickly tap your finger over the body area just below your first joint. Remember to keep the wrist of the tapping hand loose and relaxed.
- Direct percussion uses the hand or fingertip to directly tap a body area. This method is used to find tender spots and to examine a child's thorax.
- Blunt percussion uses the fist, either directly on the body area or on the back of your opposite hand, which is placed on the body area. You use this method to find tender spots. A second type of blunt percussion involves the use of the reflex hammer to create muscle contraction.

NORMAL AND ABNORMAL PERCUSSION SOUNDS

BODY AREA	SOUND	DESCRIPTION
Healthy lung	Resonance	Long, low, moderate to loud, hollow
Hyperinflated lung	Hyperresonance	Long duration, extremely loud and low-pitched, booming

NORMAL AND ABNORMAL PERCUSSION SOUNDS *(CONTINUED)*

BODY AREA	SOUND	DESCRIPTION
Pleural fluid accumulation or thickening (abnormal)	Dullness	Soft to moderately loud, thud
Abdomen	Tympany	Moderate duration, high-pitched, loud drum-like over hollow organs: stomach, intestine, bladder
	Dullness	Moderate duration, high-pitched, soft to moderately loud, thud
Muscle (normal)	Flatness	Short duration, soft, high-pitched, flat

THE PREGNANT PATIENT:
Liver, full bladder, uterus of pregnant woman

*A*SSESSMENT TECHNIQUES

Auscultation is the process of listening to the sounds different body areas produce—for example, the heart and lungs. You can hear many body sounds, such as the wheeze of the asthma sufferer, with your ear. Other sounds, such as a heart murmur, require the use of a stethoscope. With the exception of the abdomen, auscultation is the last procedure you conduct in the assessment. When assessing the abdomen, first visually inspect it and then listen for sounds. End the assessment with percussion and palpation. Otherwise, bowel sounds may be disrupted by the examination.

When using a stethoscope, observe the following procedure:

- Conduct the exam in a quiet environment.
- Use a quality instrument with bell and diaphragm with ear pieces that fit you comfortably.
- Expose the body area to which you are listening—fabric can obscure sound.
- Remind the patient not to talk during the procedure, and ask the patient to stay as still as possible.
- Warm the stethoscope head with your hand. If it is cold, the patient may jump or shiver, which will result in extraneous sounds.
- Place the stethoscope head over the body area.
- Close your eyes to eliminate any distractions.
- Listen carefully and develop a complete description of any sound you hear, including how often each occurs.

$\mathcal{P}$ERFORMING THE ASSESSMENT

In most cases, you will not have the luxury of conducting the entire assessment. In such cases, gear the assessment to the diagnosis. Use the guidelines in Chapter 1, "Health History," when conducting the assessment.

$\mathcal{C}$OMPONENTS OF THE ASSESSMENT

A full assessment is based on the patient's health history (see Chapter 1, "Health History"). You end it with an examination of all the body areas. Note any factors, including race, gender, and age, that may affect a diagnosis. Pay attention to any signs of personal distress. Signs of distress include the following:

- shortness of breath—suggesting a respiratory or cardiac problem
- wheezing or difficulty sitting still—suggesting asthma
- labored breathing—suggesting pneumonia or heart failure
- withdrawn posture, arms crossed, rapid speech, sudden hand movements—suggesting emotional distress
- limited movement, grimacing, clutching the affected area—suggesting pain

NURSE ALERT:

For severe pain, especially in the chest or abdomen, you may need to contact a physician immediately.

Assessing Elderly Patients

When assessing elderly patients, it is more important to explore current complaints than collect a past history. You may also need to modify the assessment if your patient appears confused. In that case, ask simple, direct questions and enlist the aid of someone close to the patient. Otherwise, follow the guidelines in this chapter.

Aging may reduce the body's resistance to illness, tolerance of stress, and ability to recuperate from an injury. It can also cause weakening and stiffening of the muscles; loss of hearing, sight, or the ability to smell; slowing of reflexes; and changes in vital signs.

In some cases, aging may mean a loss of intellectual and reasoning skills. Heart disease, diabetes, cataracts, and cancer are more prevalent among older patients.

It's also important to bear in mind that the elderly patient may be on many different medications. You should always watch such a patient for adverse drug reactions and interactions.

When you assess elderly patients, follow these guidelines:
- Always be respectful of the patient. Establish whether or not the patient is comfortable with conversing on a first-name basis.
- Be sure the patient can understand and follow your explanations and instructions. If not, speak slowly and simply.
- Be patient—the elderly patient may take longer to answer your questions or respond to your suggestions.
- Make sure the patient doesn't have a hearing problem. On the other hand, don't automatically raise your voice.
- Some elderly patients may have to move slowly and will have trouble getting from one position to another during the assessment. Allow them extra time.
- Watch for evidence that the patient is beginning to have difficulty taking care of himself or herself.
- Watch for evidence that the patient is not eating properly.
- Learn to identify the symptoms of age-specific diseases, such as osteoporosis and Parkinson's disease.
- Observe the patient for signs of depression. If an ordinarily neat patient begins to show up for appointments in disarray, depression may be the underlying fac-

tor. Depression can also cause mood swings, irritability, and difficulty paying attention.

- If you observe confusion in the patient, do not assume that it results from changes in the brain. Drugs, poor eating habits, dehydration, and even a change in surrounding and routines can all cause confusion in elderly people.
- Maintain a positive attitude toward normal changes of aging.

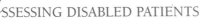

ASSESSING DISABLED PATIENTS

When assessing disabled patients, make any necessary adjustments. For example, a mute patient should be given a written questionnaire. Or, you may need a sign interpreter for a deaf patient. Use simple, direct sentences and questions with an intellectually impaired patient. In any case, it is helpful to have a close friend or relative attend the visit with the patient.

When assessing such a patient, observe the following:
- Adapt your interaction with the patient to his or her abilities.
- Establish to what extent the patient can be a participant in the assessment before you begin. A severely mentally disabled patient may not be able to participate at all. Other patients may require special assistance.
- Be sensitive to the patient's needs and emotional state.
- Pay attention to the patient's feelings about the disability and about the assessment itself.
- Ascertain the patient's level of independence.

TRANSCULTURAL CONSIDERATIONS

Do not confuse cultural differences with abnormal behavior. Before drawing any conclusions, try to get a feel for cultural differences.

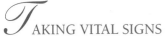

TAKING VITAL SIGNS

The taking of vital signs is fundamental to the physical assessment. Specifically, you check the patient's pulse, respiration, temperature, and blood pressure. Vital signs allow you to establish baseline values for the patient and record changes in the patient's health status. It is preferable to take the signs at once because variations from the norm can indicate possible problems with the patient's health.

A single measure of a vital sign is less reliable than multiple measurements. Ask patients what is normal for them.

If a patient shows an abnormal pattern in a vital sign, make sure that you don't show any apprehension or concern. You should explore any change in vital signs.

NURSE ALERT:
If you take a reading that you think is inaccurate, repeat it. If it still seems inaccurate, have another nurse perform the reading. If you still question the reading, try using a different instrument to check its validity. Explain why you are repeating the measurement.

MEASURING HEIGHT AND WEIGHT

Keeping track of your patient's height and weight is as important as assessing his or her vital signs. When measurements are taken regularly, they help you track the patient's growth and development. If, for example, the patient exhibits a sudden weight loss, this alerts you to the possible onset of illness.

You will also use height and weight in calculating doses of drugs. They are also a way of measuring the success of drugs, fluid, or nutrients administered I.V.

MEASURING PULSE

To take the pulse, you generally use the wrist. If the patient's wrist is injured, or if the patient has diabetes or vascular insufficiency, you will also check all the peripheral pulses to make sure that circulation is normal.

When taking the pulse, palpate the artery for 60 seconds while applying gentle compression. It's less accurate to count for 15 seconds and multiply by 4 because you are likely to miss any abnormalities in heart rate or rhythm.

NURSE ALERT:
If you must use the carotid artery, be extremely careful with the amount of pressure you place on the artery. Too much pressure can trigger reflex bradycardia. Never press on both carotid arteries at once because you can disrupt circulation to the brain.

When taking an infant's or a toddler's pulse, you can either auscultate the apical pulse or palpate the carotid, femoral, atrial, or brachial pulse. You can also take the pulse by watching the movement of the anterior fontanelle.

MEASURING BLOOD PRESSURE

When taking blood pressure, observe the following:
- Check that the patient has not exercised or eaten in the past 30 minutes.
- Make sure that the patient is relaxed.
- Check that the cuff is the right size for the patient. If the cuff is too small, the blood pressure will be falsely elevated; if the cuff is too large, the blood pressure will be falsely lowered.
- Make sure that the bladder is centered over the brachial artery.
- Keep the patient's arm level with the heart by supporting it.
- Listen for pulse sounds as you slowly open the air valve:
  - The beginning of a clear, soft tapping that increases to a thud or loud tap. This is the systolic presssure sound.
  - The change of the tapping to a soft, swishing sound
  - The return of the clear tapping sound
  - A muffled, blowing sound. This is the first diastolic sound. If your patient is a child or physically active adult, this reading is the most accurate reading of diastolic pressure.
  - The disappearance of the muffled, blowing sound. This is the second diastolic sound.

It is more accurate to record the blood pressure readings at the systolic pressure, the first diastolic and the second diastolic sound—for example—110/72/70, although this is not usually done in daily practice.

ASSESSING RESPIRATORY PATTERNS

When assessing respiration, be sure to ascertain the rate, rhythm, and depth.

RESPIRATORY PATTERNS

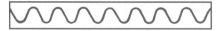

Eupnea
Normal respiratory rate and rhythm

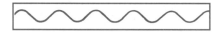

Tachypnea
Increased respiratory rate

Bradypnea
Slow but regular respirations

Apnea
Periodic absence of breathing

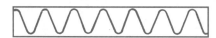

Hyperventilation
Deeper respirations, but at normal rate

ASSESSING REPIRATORY PATTERNS *(CONTINUED)*

RESPIRATORY PATTERNS

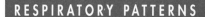

CHEYNE-STOKES
Gradually quickening and deepening respirations, alternating with slower respirations and periods of apnea

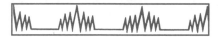

BIOT'S
Faster and deeper than normal respirations of equal depth punctuated with abrupt pauses

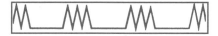

KUSSMAUL'S
Faster and deeper than normal respirations without pauses

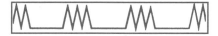

APNEUSTIC
Respirations with prolonged, gasping inspirations followed by very short, inefficient expiration

$\mathscr{C}$hapter 3. Head-to-Toe Physical Assessment

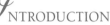

$\mathscr{I}$NTRODUCTION

SEE TEXT PAGES

This chapter contains a collection of charts that will serve as a guide to assessing the patient from head to toe.

ASSESSMENT TECHNIQUES: HEAD AND NECK

ASSESSMENT	NORMAL FINDINGS	DEVIATIONS FROM NORMAL
Inspect hair, scalp color, and condition.	Normal color; normal texture; full distribution over scalp; scalp pink, smooth, mobile, and free of lesions **THE ELDERLY:** May have thin hair.	Thinning or thickening of the hair—endocrine disorders or side effects from medications; dandruff; dull, coarse, brittle hair; nits
Palpate from the forehead to the posterior triangle of the neck for posterior cervical lymph nodes.	Symmetrical, rounded normocephalic head, positioned at midline, with no lumps or ridges	Note unusual asymmetry, changes in head size, enlarged or painful lymph glands
Palpate around the ears, under the chin, and in the anterior triangle for anterior cervical lymph nodes.	Nonpalpable lymph nodes or small, soft, round, mobile lymph nodes without tenderness	Note the location, size, consistency, tenderness, temperature, and mobility of any enlarged nodes

ASSESSMENT TECHNIQUES: HEAD AND NECK (CONTINUED)

ASSESSMENT	NORMAL FINDINGS	DEVIATIONS FROM NORMAL
Auscultate the carotid arteries.	No bruit on auscultation	Bruit—area of turbulent blood flow
Palpate the trachea.	Straight, midline	Deviation from the midline
Use only one finger to palpate the suprasternal notch.	Palpable pulsations with even rhythm	Abnormal aortic arch pulsations
Palpate the supraclavicular area.	Nonpalpable lymph nodes	Enlarged lymph nodes
Gently palpate the left and then the right carotid artery using the index and middle fingers.	Equal pulse amplitude and rhythm	Unequal pulse amplitude and rhythm

!

NURSE ALERT:
Do not palpate both sides of the anterior neck at the same time. If you accidentally press on both carotid arteries, you may interrupt blood flow to the brain.

ASSESSMENT TECHNIQUES: HEAD AND NECK (*CONTINUED*)

ASSESSMENT	NORMAL FINDINGS	DEVIATIONS FROM NORMAL
Use the pads of your fingers to palpate the thyroid gland; inside the sternocleidomastoid muscle and below the cricoid and thyroid cartilage.	Thin, mobile thyroid isthmus; nonpalpable thyroid lobes	Enlarged or tender thyroid, nodules **!** **NURSE ALERT:** If you find an enlarged thyroid, auscultate for bruits.
Have patient shrug the shoulders against resistance applied by your hands.	Normal range of motion, equal range and strength **THE ELDERLY** May have difficulty tilting the head. Only move the head to the point of discomfort.	Loss of full range of motion
Have patient touch chin to the chest and to each shoulder, touch ear to each shoulder, and tilt head back	Equal strength and movement	Asymmetrical strength or movement
Have patient push left cheek and then right cheek against your hand.	Equal strength and movement	Asymmetrical strength or movement

ASSESSMENT TECHNIQUES: HEAD AND NECK (CONTINUED)

ASSESSMENT	NORMAL FINDINGS	DEVIATIONS FROM NORMAL
Inspect patient's face.	Symmetrical facial features	Edema, lesions, or deformities
Have patient smile, wrinkle forehead, puff cheeks.	Symmetrical in all actions	Asymmetrical in any action
Inspect nose.	Symmetrical and non-deviated; tissue pink and nontender	Edema, deformity, nasal discharge, discoloration, flared nostrils, redness, swelling **NURSE ALERT:** Note color of any mucus.
Alternate holding one nostril shut while patient breathes through the other.	Equal functioning, both passages clear	Inability to breathe through either or both nostrils
Support the patient's head with your free hand and use an ophthalmoscope handle with a nasal attachment to inspect internal nostrils. **NURSE ALERT:** Don't use an ophthalmoscope handle with a nasal attachment on an infant or young child. It is too sharp. Use a flashlight for illumination instead.	Pink mucosa **THE PREGNANT PATIENT:** Nasal mucosa may be mildly swollen.	Inflamed, swollen mucosa; polyps

ASSESSMENT TECHNIQUES: HEAD AND NECK (*CONTINUED*)

ASSESSMENT	NORMAL FINDINGS	DEVIATIONS FROM NORMAL
Gently palpate the nose.	Symmetrical, smooth	Edema, bumps, tenderness, asymmetry
Percuss and palpate the sinuses.	No tenderness	Tenderness. If tender, transilluminate the sinuses.

!

NURSE ALERT:
Prior to age 8, the frontal sinus is too small to percuss or palpate.

Have patient open and close mouth while you palpate temporomandibular joints with your middle three fingers.	Smooth, quiet movement; bones aligned	Misalignment, tenderness, clicking

ASSESSMENT TECHNIQUES: HEAD AND NECK (CONTINUED)

ASSESSMENT	NORMAL FINDINGS	DEVIATIONS FROM NORMAL
Inspect interior structure of mouth with tongue depressor and penlight.	Pink mucosa and gingiva	Inflammation, edema

NURSE ALERT:
Have the patient remove any dental prosthetics. Wear gloves.

THE PREGNANT PATIENT
In the pregnant patient, you may find the gingiva to be swollen.

TRANSCULTURAL CONSIDERTIONS:
The mucosa of dark-skinned patients is bluish. This pigmentation is normal.

THE CHILD
A child may have as many as 20 baby teeth. The emergence of baby teeth begins at approximately 6 months. Baby teeth are replaced by secondary teeth between the ages of 6 and 12.

ASSESSMENT TECHNIQUES: HEAD AND NECK (CONTINUED)

ASSESSMENT	NORMAL FINDINGS	DEVIATIONS FROM NORMAL
Inspect the tongue and palates. ! **NURSE ALERT:** Use this to check hydration in children.	Pink, moist; without ulcers or lesions	Inflammation; lesions; dry, cracked tongue; coated tongue; red inflamed tongue; gingiva on palate
Have patient stick out tongue.	Midline	Cannot hold tongue straight
Have patient stick out tongue and say "Ahh."	Soft palate and uvula rise symmetrically; pink, midline uvula; both tonsils behind pillars	Asymmetry of structures; swollen, inflamed tonsils
Lightly touch back of tongue to test gag reflex. ! **NURSE ALERT:** If your patient is nauseated, you may want to skip this assessment.	Patient gags; if swallowing is intact, usually gag reflex is present	No gag reflex ! **NURSE ALERT:** Perform when problem suspected with cranial nerves 9 and 10.

ASSESSMENT TECHNIQUES: HEAD AND NECK *(CONTINUED)*

ASSESSMENT	NORMAL FINDINGS	DEVIATIONS FROM NORMAL
Have patient push against tongue depressor with each side of tongue.	Symmetrical movement and strength	Asymmetry, loss of taste ! **NURSE ALERT:** If patient reports loss of taste, test with cotton swabs dipped in vinegar, sugar, etc.
Use a test tube containing a familiar substance, like coffee, to test smell. ! **NURSE ALERT:** Have patient close eyes.	Correctly identifies substance	Unable to identify common substance
Test visual acuity using Snellen eye chart. **THE CHILD:** A young child's vision may be 20/30.	20/20 vision; patients over age 40 may have reduced near vision.	Hesitancy, squinting, vision poorer than 20/30—suggest patient visit an ophthalmologist

ASSESSMENT TECHNIQUES: HEAD AND NECK (CONTINUED)

ASSESSMENT	NORMAL FINDINGS	DEVIATIONS FROM NORMAL
Have patient read newsprint aloud held at a distance of 12 to 14 in (30.5 to 35.5 cm)	Normal near vision	Abnormal near vision—suggest patient visit an ophthalmologist

NURSE ALERT:
Make sure patient wears any corrective lenses.

NURSE ALERT:
If patient is illiterate, use Snellen E chart.

ASSESSMENT	NORMAL FINDINGS	DEVIATIONS FROM NORMAL
Have patient identify pattern of colored dots on a special color plate.	Identifies pattern; accurate color perception	Cannot identify pattern

NURSE ALERT:
It's very important to diagnose color blindness in a child as early as possible. This gives the child ample time to learn to compensate and alerts parents and other caretakers.

ASSESSMENT TECHNIQUES: HEAD AND NECK (CONTINUED)

ASSESSMENT	NORMAL FINDINGS	DEVIATIONS FROM NORMAL
Perform six cardinal positions of gaze test.	Bilaterally equal eye movement; no nystagmus	Nystagmus **NURSE ALERT:** Refer any patient who cannot pass this test to an ophthamlologist.
Perform cover/uncover test.	Eyes steady; no jerking or wandering eye movement	Wandering, jerking **NURSE ALERT:** Refer any patient who cannot pass this test to an ophthalmologist.
Perform corneal light reflex test.	Eyes steadily fixed on an object. Bilateral corneal light reflection	Eyes not parallel when fixed on an object **NURSE ALERT:** Refer any patient who cannot pass this test to an ophthalmologist.

ASSESSMENT TECHNIQUES: HEAD AND NECK (CONTINUED)

ASSESSMENT	NORMAL FINDINGS	DEVIATIONS FROM NORMAL
Test peripheral vision.	Normal vision laterally, above, down, and medially, **THE ELDERLY** Patient may have decreased peripheral vision.	Vision deviates from 50 degrees from top, 60 degrees medially, 70 degrees downward, 110 degrees laterally; detects only large defects in peripheral vision
Inspect external eye structures.	Clear, symmetrical eyes; even eyelashes **THE ELDERLY** May have few eyelashes, dull eyes. **TRANSCULTURAL CONSIDERATIONS** Asian patients may have eyelids with epicanthal folds.	Cloudy eyes with nystagmus, asymmetry, lid lag, bulging, edema, redness, outward or inward-turning lids, styes, edema, scaling, lesions, unequally distributed eyelashes, eyelashes curve inward, reddened lacrimal apparatus

ASSESSMENT TECHNIQUES: HEAD AND NECK (CONTINUED)

ASSESSMENT	NORMAL FINDINGS	DEVIATIONS FROM NORMAL
Palpate lacrimal apparatus to check tear ducts.	Nontender, pink; without drainage or lumps	Tenderness, masses, too much tearing, drainage **NURSE ALERT:** Culture any drainage.
Examine conjunctiva and sclera. **NURSE ALERT:** Wash hands between examining each eye.	Pink conjunctiva with no drainage; clear sclera **THE ELDERLY** May have pinguecula. **TRANSCULTURAL CONSIDERATIONS** Small spots on sclera are normal in dark-skinned patients.	Edema, drainage, hyperemic blood vessels, inflammation, conjunctivitis, color changes in sclera, scleral icterus

ASSESSMENT TECHNIQUES: HEAD AND NECK (CONTINUED)

ASSESSMENT	NORMAL FINDINGS	DEVIATIONS FROM NORMAL
Shine penlight across eye to examine cornea, iris, and anterior chamber.	Clear, transparent **THE ELDERLY** Cornea may have thin, graying ring. **TRANSCULTURAL CONSIDERATIONS** A gray-blue cornea is normal in dark-skinned patients.	Clouding of cornea, portion of iris does not illuminate
Check pupils.	PERRLA: pupils equal, round, reactive to light and accommodation **THE ELDERLY** After age 85 pupils may not react to accommodation.	Asymmetry in size, asymmetrical reaction to light or its absence, fixed pupils, dilated or constricted pupils
Use ophthalmoscope to check red reflex.	Clearly defined orange-red glow	Absence of red reflex—indicative of opacity and clouding

ASSESSMENT TECHNIQUES: HEAD AND NECK (CONTINUED)

ASSESSMENT	NORMAL FINDINGS	DEVIATIONS FROM NORMAL
Check ears.	Line up with eyes, same color as face, symmetrical and proportional to face	Asymmetry, lesions, redness, hard-packed ear wax, drainage, nodules

THE ELDERLY
Reduced adipose tissue and hardened cartilage

TRANSCULTURAL CONSIDERATIONS
Ear wax is yellow in light-skinned patients and dark orange or brown in dark-skinned patients.

Palpate ear and mastoid process.	Absence of pain, tenderness, and swelling	Tenderness, pain, edema, lesions, nodules

NURSE ALERT:
If otitis externa, tenderness, or edema is present, be careful with the otoscope—you may be unable to use it.

ASSESSMENT TECHNIQUES: HEAD AND NECK (CONTINUED)

ASSESSMENT	NORMAL FINDINGS	DEVIATIONS FROM NORMAL
Check hearing in each ear by whispering or holding a ticking watch to the ear.	Normal hearing (whisper from 1 to 2 ft; tick from 5 in) **!** **NURSE ALERT:** Note the distance at which you perform the test.	Loss of hearing
Weber's test with tuning fork.	Vibrations heard equally in both ears	Sound heard best in ear with conductive hearing loss
Rinne test with tuning fork.	Equal period of hearing in front of ear and on mastoid process	Conductive or sensorineural hearing loss; vibrations heard longer on mastoid process or front of ear

ASSESSMENT TECHNIQUES: POSTERIOR THORAX

ASSESSMENT	NORMAL FINDINGS	DEVIATIONS FROM NORMAL
Examine the back.	Normal skin tone, symmetry of structure, shoulder height, and inhalation	Asymmetry, accessory muscle use, scoliosis

ASSESSMENT TECHNIQUES: POSTERIOR THORAX *(CONTINUED)*

ASSESSMENT	NORMAL FINDINGS	DEVIATIONS FROM NORMAL
Examine the antero-posterior and lateral thorax. **THE CHILD** Measure chest circumference at nipples.	2:1 relationship between lateral and anteroposterior diameter **THE ELDERLY** Diameter ratio may normally increase.	Increased diameter indicative of pulmonary disease
Palpate the spine.	Straight alignment Firm, symmetrical	Abnormal alignment, lesions, tenderness, asymmetrical muscles, pain
Palpate the posterior thorax.	Normal, smooth	Lesions, lumps, pain, inflammation, abnormalities
Percuss the costovertebral area.	Normal thud	Pain, tenderness

ASSESSMENT TECHNIQUES: POSTERIOR THORAX (*CONTINUED*)

ASSESSMENT	NORMAL FINDINGS	DEVIATIONS FROM NORMAL
Inspect respiratory function.	Symmetrical expansion and contraction	Asymmetry
Palpate as patient says "99" over and over.	Symmetrical vibration Note: Vibration varies over chest.	Increased vibration
Percuss systematically over the lung area.	Resonant over lungs and dull over diaphragm	Asymmetrical sounds, dull over lungs, hyperresonance (pulmonary disease)

THE CHILD
An infant's chest is too small for reliable percussion.

THE ELDERLY
Hyperresonant sounds possible from hyperinflation of lung tissue.

ASSESSMENT TECHNIQUES: POSTERIOR THORAX (*CONTINUED*)

ASSESSMENT	NORMAL FINDINGS	DEVIATIONS FROM NORMAL
Percuss each side of posterior thorax for diaphragmatic excursion.	1¼ to 2¼ in excursion **NURSE ALERT:** The right side of the diaphragm is usually higher than the left.	Unequal excursion
Have patient take slow, deep breaths through mouth while you systematically auscultate the lungs. **THE CHILD** Auscultate a child first—other procedures may cause crying. **NURSE ALERT:** If the patient has a great deal of chest hair, moisten it to reduce interference.	Bronchial, vesicular, and bronchovesicular sounds **THE CHILD** A child may normally have coarser lung sounds.	Wheezing, coarse to fine crackles, rhonchi **NURSE ALERT:** Crackles may indicate congestive heart failure.

ASSESSMENT TECHNIQUES: ANTERIOR THORAX

ASSESSMENT	NORMAL FINDINGS	DEVIATIONS FROM NORMAL
Inspect anterior thoracic area.	Normal skin tone, symmetry of structures and inhalation **!** **NURSE ALERT:** Children and men breathe with their diaphragm muscles, adult women breathe with their upper chest.	Abnormal skin tone, accessory muscle use, asymmetry, deformity, lifts, heaves, or thrusts, point of maximum impulse visible **!** **NURSE ALERT:** Children and very thin patients may normally have visible point of maximum impulse.
Palpate anterior thorax.	No tenderness or lesions	Lesions, lumps, pain, left and right symmetry
Inspect respiratory excursion.	Symmetrical expansion and contraction	Asymmetrical expansion and contraction

ASSESSMENT TECHNIQUES: ANTERIOR THORAX (CONTINUED)

ASSESSMENT	NORMAL FINDINGS	DEVIATIONS FROM NORMAL
Palpate as patient repeats "99" over and over.	Resonant lung fields, dullness over bony structures	Dullness over lung fields, abnormal sounds over bony structures
THE CHILD Unreliable in an infant.	**THE ELDERLY** May have hyperresonant sounds.	
Perform a breast exam. **NURSE ALERT:** Have a patient with large, pendulous breasts lean forward.	Soft, symmetrical breasts, symmetrical nipples **THE PREGNANT PATIENT** Breasts are swollen, nipples dark, areola dark, may have purple streaks.	Asymmetry, abnormal hair growth, lesions, lumps, nodes, thickening; cracks, fissures, blisters, inflammation, pain, etc. **NURSE ALERT:** Culture any nipple discharge.
With patient at 45 degree angle, inspect jugular veins.	No pulsation	Distended, changes in bounding pulse

ASSESSMENT TECHNIQUES: ANTERIOR THORAX *(CONTINUED)*

ASSESSMENT	NORMAL FINDINGS	DEVIATIONS FROM NORMAL
Palpate precordium.	Point of maximum impulse at apical area	Shift in point of maximum impulse indicates abnormal changes in left ventricle
Auscultate for heart sounds.	S_1 and S_2, normal rhythm, pulse rate normal for age	Extra heart sounds, murmurs, rubs **THE CHILD** A child may have benign heart murmurs.

ASSESSMENT TECHNIQUES: ABDOMEN

ASSESSMENT	NORMAL FINDINGS	DEVIATIONS FROM NORMAL
Inspect abdomen.	Normal contour for body type and age, normal skin color	Asymmetry, bulges, visible growths, abnormal color, rash, visible peristaltic waves, hernia, lesions

ASSESSMENT TECHNIQUES: ABDOMEN *(CONTINUED)*

ASSESSMENT	NORMAL FINDINGS	DEVIATIONS FROM NORMAL
Systematically auscultate abdomen for up to 5 minutes in all four quadrants	Normal bowel sounds in all areas	Bruits, other abnormal sounds; hyperactive sounds in one area followed by absent sound

NURSE ALERT:
Auscultate before percussion or palpation. If you perform either procedure first, you may generate abnormal sounds or rupture an aneurysm.

Percuss on left and right side from just below breast to midclavicular line.	Dull over liver, tympanic over abdomen	Abnormal sounds

NURSE ALERT:
You may not feel the liver border if the patient has gas in the colon or congestion in the right lower lung.

ASSESSMENT TECHNIQUES: ABDOMEN (*CONTINUED*)

ASSESSMENT	NORMAL FINDINGS	DEVIATIONS FROM NORMAL
Systematically palpate abdomen, moving from upper to lower areas in each quadrant. **NURSE ALERT:** It helps a ticklish patient to place a hand over yours while you palpate.	Soft, nontender symmetrical abdomen	Tenderness, masses, pain, bladder distention **NURSE ALERT:** Examine any painful area last to prevent the patient from tensing to guard the area.
Palpate the liver.	Often nonpalpable; if edge palpable, smooth, nontender	Mushy, enlarged, lumps
Palpate the spleen.	Nonpalpable	Palpable (enlarged)
Palpate femoral groin pulse. **THE CHILD** This is an important pulse point in children.	Symmetrical, strong	Asymmetrical, weak or absent **NURSE ALERT:** Absent pulse with blue extremities is a clinical emergency.

ASSESSMENT TECHNIQUES: UPPER EXTREMITIES

ASSESSMENT	NORMAL FINDINGS	DEVIATIONS FROM NORMAL
Inspect the upper extremities.	Normal, uniform skin color and texture, symmetrical muscle mass, good skin turgor	Abnormal color or texture, lesions, dryness, asymmetrical muscle mass, poor skin turgor
THE CHILD Skin turgor on the upper extremities and chest is important for identifying dehydration in infants and young children.	**THE ELDERLY** Skin may be dry and thin with deficient turgor.	
Have patient turn palms up and down with arms extended.	Steady hands, symmetrical movement	Tremors, pronator drift, unable to follow instructions
Have patient push forearms up and down against your hand.	Symmetrical strength and movement	Asymmetry when comparing left to right
Inspect and palpate all joints.	Normal range of motion	Stiffness, edema, enlarged joint, redness, pain with movement, limited range of motion

ASSESSMENT TECHNIQUES: UPPER EXTREMITIES *(CONTINUED)*

ASSESSMENT	NORMAL FINDINGS	DEVIATIONS FROM NORMAL
Palpate hands for temperature.	Warm, moist, symmetrical	Cool, clammy skin or warm, dry skin; asymmetry
Palpate brachial pulses.	Right and left equal	Decreased pulse strength, thready pulse, difference between right and left pulse
Inspect fingernails.	Color, shape, and condition normal, good capillary refill	Broken and cracked nails, pitting, clubbing, cyanosis, decreased capillary refill
Have patient squeeze two of your fingers with each fist.	Symmetry in hand strength	Asymmetry

ASSESSMENT TECHNIQUES: LOWER EXTREMITIES

ASSESSMENT	NORMAL FINDINGS	DEVIATIONS FROM NORMAL
Inspect lower extremities.	Even skin color and texture, symmetrical muscle mass, hair and nail growth	Abnormal color, lesions, dryness, hair loss, bruises, varicosity, edema, fungal toe nails, asymmetrical muscle mass

ASSESSMENT TECHNIQUES: LOWER EXTREMITIES (CONTINUED)

ASSESSMENT	NORMAL FINDINGS	DEVIATIONS FROM NORMAL
Palpate for pitting edema between knee and ankle and in foot.	No edema	Pitting edema present— grade according to scale
Palpate posterior tibial area and dorsalis pedis.	Symmetrical pulse, skin temperature	Asymmetrical, weak, or absent pulse; skin temperature decreases **NURSE ALERT:** If any pulse is abnormal, check the popliteal pulse.
Perform the straight leg test on each leg.	Normal movement **THE ELDERLY** May have difficulty with this test.	Pain with extension **NURSE ALERT:** Help a patient with difficulty extending by steadying leg.

ASSESSMENT TECHNIQUES: LOWER EXTREMITIES (CONTINUED)

ASSESSMENT	NORMAL FINDINGS	DEVIATIONS FROM NORMAL
Palpate hip with abduction and adduction.	No crepitus	Crepitus

THE CHILD
Use Ortolani's maneuver on an infant.

Have patient raise each thigh against your hand; push tibial area out against your hand; pull calf back against your hand.	Symmetrical strength	Weak or asymmetrical strength

THE CHILD
Test strength by having child hop on each leg.

SUGGESTED READINGS

Anderson, F. D., and J. Malone. "Taking Blood Pressure." Nursing94 24 (November 1994): 34–39.

Flory, C. "Perfecting the Art of Skin Assessment." RN 55 (June 1992): 22–27.

Hartrick, G., and A. E. Lindsey. "Family Nursing Assessment: Meeting the Challenge of Health Promotion." Journal of Advanced Nursing 20 (July 1994): 85–91.

Jensen, L., and M. Allen. "Wellness—The Dialectic of Illness." Image, Journal of Nursing Scholarship 2 (Fall 1993): 220–224.

SECTION II: RESPIRATORY ASSESSMENT

Chapter 4: Anatomy and Physiology

▽   ▽   ▽   ▽   ▽   ▽   ▽

ANATOMY

SEE TEXT PAGES

Anatomy of the respiratory tract includes the:
- Structures of the nasal cavity, where outside air is drawn into the body
- Conducting airways, from the trachea into the lungs
- Acinus, where the exchange of oxygen occurs

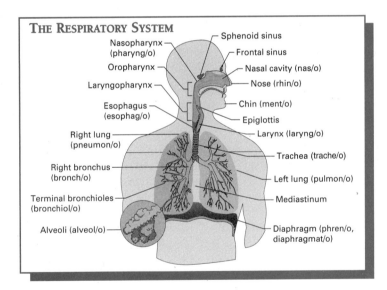

THE RESPIRATORY SYSTEM

Nasopharynx (pharyng/o)
Oropharynx
Laryngopharynx
Esophagus (esophag/o)
Right lung (pneumon/o)
Right bronchus (bronch/o)
Terminal bronchioles (bronchiol/o)
Alveoli (alveol/o)

Sphenoid sinus
Frontal sinus
Nasal cavity (nas/o)
Nose (rhin/o)
Chin (ment/o)
Epiglottis
Larynx (laryng/o)
Trachea (trache/o)
Left lung (pulmon/o)
Mediastinum
Diaphragm (phren/o, diaphragmat/o)

From the nostrils through the bronchioles, the air-conducting passages are lined with ciliated mucous membrane to warm, humidify, and filter the incoming air. A network of blood vessels underlying the mucosa warms the air, while moisture from this mucosa blanket humidifies it. Filtration is begun by hairs in the vestibule, which trap larger particles, and is continued by the mucosa blanket, which traps smaller particles.

The cells in the conducting airways are primarily pseudo-stratified, ciliated, columnar epithelial cells, interspersed with goblet and serous cells. The epithelial surface is covered by mucus secreted by goblet and serous cells.

Structures of the nasal cavity include:
- Nose. The anterior naris (nostril) is the means through which air enters the nose, passing through the hair-lined vestibule into the nasopharynx. The upper third of the nose is supported by bone; the lower two thirds are supported by cartilage.
- Turbinates. Bony structures within the nasal cavity are covered by a mucosa blanket with many blood vessels. These structures increase the surface area available for warming, humidifying, and cleansing air as it enters the nose.
- Sinuses. Air-filled extensions of the nasal cavity are also lined with mucosa, along with cilia to move secretions through the nasal cavity.

Structures of the tracheobronchial tree include:
- Pharynx. This tubular passageway (the throat) connects the nasal cavity to the larynx. The tonsils are located in the pharynx and act to filter and destroy invading microorganisms that have not been trapped in the nasal area.
- Larynx. This passageway, between the pharynx and the trachea, is composed of a series of rings of cartilage, united by muscles. It contains:
  - Vocal cords: the lower two folds of the larynx that produce sound when air is drawn over them
  - Glottis: a triangular space between the vocal cords, opening into the trachea and forming the division between the upper and lower respiratory tract
  - Epiglottis: a leaf-shaped structure at the entrance to the larynx, which closes when the larynx rises during swallowing to direct food to the esophagus
- Trachea. This 5-inch passageway is supported by U-shaped cartilaginous rings. The opening in the U is toward the posterior, where the trachea appears flattened. It lies immediately in front of the esophagus, and connects the larynx to the bronchi. The point at which the trachea branches into the bronchi is the carina.
- Bronchi. These passageways, composed of cartilage and smooth muscle, are the main branches of the tracheobronchial tree. They are not symmetrical: the left branch is longer and narrower and branches from the trachea at

a more acute angle than the right bronchi. The bronchi
continue to subdivide through approximately 23 levels
until they reach the acinus. Beginning at the carina, the
branching continues through the lobar (or first level)
bronchi to the segmental bronchi to the terminal bronchiole, which is the lowest level before reaching the alveoli.

- Acinus. The acinus is beyond the terminal bronchiole,
and is the location in which the gas exchange takes
place. It is sometimes called the primary lobule or atri-
um, and consists of:
  - Respiratory bronchioles: cavities with small alveoli (air
  sacs) around the walls
  - Alveolar ducts: cavities completely lined with alveoli
  - Terminal alveolar sacs: the final structure of lung that
  contains clusters of individual alveoli
- Alveoli. Small sacs, separated from their neighbors by
thin septum. Small openings in the septum, called pores
of Kohn, allow air to pass between sacs. Alveolar walls
are only as deep as one layer of cells. There are approximately 30 million alveoli in a lung, providing the surface
area for the exchange of gases. Each alveolus is lined
with surfactant, a substance that helps maintain the
structure of the alveolus during the respiratory cycle. The
final filtration of air occurs in the alveoli, where
microphages ingest microorganisms that have escaped
trapping by the defense mechanisms located in the first
portions of the tracheobronchial tree.
- Lungs. The lungs themselves are elastic, spongy, cone-
shaped organs, located in the thoracic cavity. The thoracic cavity is formed by the ribs, sternum, and vertebrae
and is separated from the abdominal cavity by the
diaphragm.

Each lung has an apex and a base and is divided into
lobes. The right lung is larger, and has three lobes, while
the left has only two lobes. The lobes divide into segments corresponding to the segmented bronchi. There
are ten segments in the right lung, nine in the left lung.
Nerves, lymphatics, and blood vessels, as well as the
bronchi, enter the lung at the hilus, forming the root of
the lung.

The lungs are covered in visceral pleura, a thin sheet of
collagen and elastic tissue. Pleural fluid, lying between
the visceral pleura and the parietal pleura, which lines
the thoracic cavity, allows the two surfaces to slide

against one another and maintain unbroken contact. Each lung is enclosed in a separate pleural sac, with no connection between the sacs. Pressure is greater within the lungs and in the atmosphere than in pleural spaces. This, therefore, creates a partial vacuum, holding the lungs against the thoracic cavity walls, allowing for ventilation and preventing lung collapse.

PHYSIOLOGY

Respiratory functioning involves three primary processes: ventilation (the movement of air into and out of the lungs), internal respiration, and external respiration. External respiration is the exchange of gases between the alveoli and blood cells in the capillaries located in the acini of the lungs, while internal respiration is the exchange of gases between blood cells in capillaries throughout the body and the cells in the body's various organs and tissues.

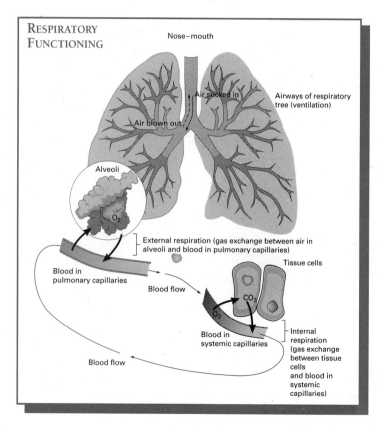

RESPIRATORY FUNCTIONING

Nose–mouth

Air sucked in

Airways of respiratory tree (ventilation)

Air blown out

Alveoli

O_2

External respiration (gas exchange between air in alveoli and blood in pulmonary capillaries)

Blood in pulmonary capillaries

Blood flow

Tissue cells

CO_2

O_2

Blood in systemic capillaries

Internal respiration (gas exchange between tissue cells and blood in systemic capillaries)

Blood flow

Additionally, other processes are required to complete the respiratory cycle. These include the adequate perfusion of blood into the structures of the lung, adequate intake of air into the lungs to sustain the process, and accurate neurologic control of respiratory function.

Control of the respiratory function is managed by the pons and medulla. The medulla transmits basic rhythm signals via its inspiratory and expiratory areas, while the pons sends signals to the medulla's inspiratory area to stop and start the rhythm. These functions can be overridden by voluntary control arising in the cerebral cortex.

A fail-safe mechanism is invoked when a certain level of carbon dioxide is reached in the blood. At that point, the medulla's inspiratory area is stimulated again and the ventilation process is resumed. The normal process can also be overridden by chemical stimuli. When the levels of oxygen and carbon dioxide shift, the medulla responds by altering the activity of inspiratory and expiratory areas. Body temperature can also cause a change in the normal inspiration and expiration process.

Ventilation is divided into two processes: inhalation and exhalation. The process of inhalation is generally an active one, while exhalation is generally passive.

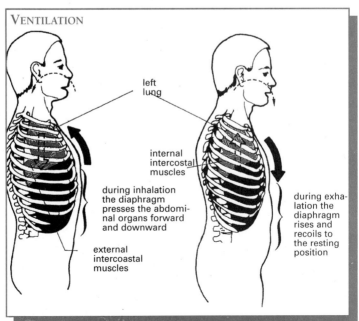

VENTILATION

left lung

internal intercostal muscles

during inhalation the diaphragm presses the abdominal organs forward and downward

external intercoastal muscles

during exhalation the diaphragm rises and recoils to the resting position

Inhalation, or inspiration, is the movement of air into the lungs caused by an imbalance in pressure between the air outside and inside the lung. During inhalation, the available volume of the lungs increases, causing the pressure inside to be less than the pressure outside. This expansion of lung volume is caused by the contraction of the diaphragm, which lowers the dome of the diaphragm and the contraction of the external intercostal muscles, which pull the ribs up and out, and raise the sternum.

When the pressures are balanced, inhalation stops and exhalation, or expiration, begins. The muscles relax, a passive process, and air rushes out of the lungs into the atmosphere, where the pressure is lower.

The air drawn into the lungs is transferred first from alveoli to blood cells in the capillaries of the lungs and then from these blood cells into other cells in every part of the body.

External respiration is the actual exchange of oxygen across the alveolar-capillary membrane. This membrane is also known as the respiratory membrane, or blood-air barrier. Oxygen and carbon dioxide pass through the respiratory membrane with differing diffusion rates, allowing for the exchange.

Internal respiration is the delivery of gases to cells throughout the body by the blood cells to which oxygen was transferred via external respiration. This process, also called cell respiration, allows for the exchange of oxygen and waste products using a mechanism similar to that of external respiration.

THE ELDERLY:
In the elderly patient, you will see an atrophy of the muscles and mucosa of the respiratory tract. Atrophy of the mucosa may decrease the efficiency of filtration, humidification, and heating processes. Atrophy of the respiratory muscles may cause difficulties in the ventilation process. As the lungs settle into the body and the diameter of the lungs is reduced, there is less alveolar space in which external respiration can occur.

Chapter 5: Subjective Data Collection

▽ ▽ ▽ ▽ ▽ ▽ ▽

INTRODUCTION

SEE TEXT PAGES

When conducting a history interview for patients suffering from respiratory distress, it's important, as with other conditions, to strike a balance between getting the necessary information and unduly stressing the patient.

Begin the interview by introducing yourself to the patient. Explain how the questions will be organized. If the patient has come with a specific complaint, explore that area first, and follow up with some general questions. If the patient has come for preventive care or a nonspecific examination, explain that you will be asking general questions about family and personal history and specific questions related to respiratory functions.

The three most common complaints associated with respiratory illness or disease are cough, shortness of breath, and chest pain. They often occur together. When they do, it's important to note which symptom is causing the most distress to the patient. It's also important to note the lack of a symptom, as its absence may help to refine the assessment. The chronology of developing symptoms may also provide important clues to the patient's condition or illness. Finally, remember that these symptoms are all extremely subjective: what may be intolerable pain to one patient is minor to another.

QUESTIONS TO ASK

When investigating a specific problem, begin with a general question, such as "What brings you here today?" If basic information is provided, say, for example, "I see you are here because you are waking up in the night short of breath. Please tell me more about that."

COUGH

Coughing is the most common symptom of respiratory disease. However, some patients, especially those with chronic cough, do not consider it important enough to mention or may underreport it. When you receive negative answers about coughing, ask related questions such as "Do you have to clear your throat frequently?" or "Do you have a morning smoker's cough?"

QUESTIONS TO ASK: COUGHING

- How frequently do you experience coughing? Do you cough continually or have "coughing fits"? How long have you had the cough? Did it come on gradually or suddenly?
- Is there anything that seems to cause your coughing? What can you do to alleviate it? Are you taking any medication to suppress your cough symptoms?
- Is the coughing worse at a particular time of the day or with a particular activity?
- Does the position of your body alter your coughing? Does it make it better or worse? Is it better if you are laying down?
- Does coughing interrupt your sleeping?
- Describe the nature of your coughing. Is it a deep chest cough or is it a braying cough from the throat?
- Is it a productive cough? If you cough up sputum, what is it like? What color is it? Does it have an odor? What does it smell like? What is its texture? How much would you estimate you cough up in a day? From where does the sputum originate? Does it feel like it comes from your nasal passages or lungs?
- If you cough up blood, how much? Is it blood mixed with sputum or only blood?
- Do you experience any other symptoms when this occurs? Do you have shortness of breath? Sore throat or hoarseness? If you have a sore throat, what can you do to alleviate the problem? Do you feel any chest pain?

QUESTIONS TO ASK: SHORTNESS OF BREATH (DYSPNEA)

- Please describe your feeling of shortness of breath. Do you feel as if you cannot draw in enough air in a breath? Or, do you feel that you cannot breathe fast enough?
- Do you always feel this way or are there specific situations in which you feel out of breath? If you feel this way only occasionally, what appears to cause the problem?

- Does the feeling worsen depending on the time of day? Is it, for example, worse in the morning?
- Does a change in body position make any difference? Is the problem worse or better when you are laying down?
- Does your shortness of breath interrupt sleep? How often in a night? Do you have to sleep propped up on pillows or sitting up?
- How severe is the problem? Has it recently worsened, gradually worsened, or just started abruptly?

To help a patient gauge the severity of his or her dyspnea, use a Visual Analog Scale. It may also help to have the patient record several days of dyspnea experiences to determine if there is a common cause or a pattern to the episodes.

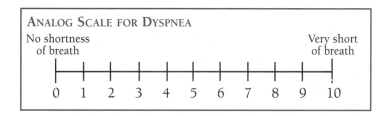

- What do you do to help ease your shortness of breath? Do you use any nasal sprays or other medications when you suffer this symptom?
- When you are short of breath, do you experience any other symptoms? Do you cough or sneeze? Do you have nasal stuffiness? If so, is it the same on both sides? Do you feel any pain? Where is the pain located? Do you experience light-headedness? Do you ever lose consciousness because of it?

CHEST PAIN

Pain is an extremely subjective finding, especially when it is not associated with obvious trauma. Be alert to signs of pain such as facial grimacing, sweating, splinting, or arrested movement.

QUESTIONS TO ASK: CHEST PAIN

- Does the pain come on suddenly, like a muscle spasm, or is it present at all times?
- Is there anything that provokes the pain? Any motion or activity? Is it worse during a particular time of the day? Does it change in time with your breathing?

- Is there anything that eases the pain? Are you taking any medication to relieve it?
- How would you describe the pain? Is it deep or superficial? Is it burning, throbbing, stabbing, or aching?
- Where is it located? Where is the center of the painful area? Does it remain localized or does it spread to other areas?
- How severe is the pain? On a scale of 1 to 10, with 10 being the worst pain you can imagine, how would you rate your pain?

NURSE ALERT:
Note that pain rated less than 5 on a scale of 1 to 10 can usually be helped by non-narcotic medication and nursing intervention measures. Pain rated greater than 5 usually requires narcotic intervention and nursing measures alone are insufficient to alleviate it.

Asking these additional general questions may help you to create a more complete picture of the patient's condition and its causes.

- Are you exposed to any kind of chemical or environmental irritant? Has this been a recent development because of, for example, a job change or move?
- Are you a smoker? Do you smoke cigarettes, a pipe, or cigars? How long have you smoked? Have you ever stopped? For how long? How many packs a day do you smoke?
- Are you exposed to second-hand smoke? Where? At home? At work? How often?
- Do you notice any pattern in your symptoms? Do they always occur in the spring, for example, or after your children start school?
- Are you taking any medications prescribed by your doctor? Over-the-counter drugs? Nasal sprays? Antihistamines?
- Do you have nosebleeds? Have you noticed anything that provokes the nosebleeds? How often do you experience nosebleeds? How long do they last? What do you do to alleviate them? Do you bruise easily on other parts of your body?
- Do you experience heart palpitations? Describe their speed, rhythm, and whether they are regular or irregular. Do they happen suddenly or gradually? How long have you been experiencing them? Is there anything that appears to provoke them? What do you do to ease the feeling?

- Have you experienced any changes in your sleeping patterns as a result of your respiratory distress? Have you recently begun to snore? Do you find yourself waking frequently in the night because of a problem in your breathing?
- When you breathe, have you noticed other noises such as wheezes or rattles? Are these prone to happen at any specific time?
- Have you noticed any facial swelling or tenderness? Are your eyes puffy or swollen when you awaken?
- Do you experience pain or tenderness in your neck or throat? Do you have "swollen glands" or feel tender lumps in your neck?
- If you are suffering from facial pain, is it the same on both sides of your face?
- Have you noticed any signs of mental confusion such as forgetfulness?
- Do you have headaches? How frequently? How would you describe the pain associated with your headaches? Where, exactly, does your head hurt?
- Do your hands tremble or shake? Are your hands and feet extremely warm or sweaty? Do you feel a tingling sensation in your hands or feet?

NURSE ALERT:
Mental confusion that can progress to the point of coma, headaches, tremors in the extremities, and warm, sweaty extremities may be indicators of hypercapnia.

- Do you find yourself yawning or sighing frequently?
- Do you have dizzy spells? How often? For how long? Is there anything that seems to cause the dizziness? What do you do to alleviate the problem?
- Have you ever experienced muscle twitches or convulsions? When? What happened, exactly?

NURSE ALERT:
Excessive sighing and yawning, dizziness, palpitations, numb or tingling extremities, and muscle twitches may be indicators of hypocapnia.

- Do others in your family have a history of respiratory problems, such as asthma or emphysema? Does anyone suffer from allergies? Has anyone had cancer, tuberculosis, or cystic fibrosis?

Chapter 6: Objective Data Collection

▽   ▽   ▽   ▽   ▽   ▽   ▽

PERFORMING THE ASSESSMENT

SEE TEXT PAGES

As you did in taking the patient's history, make every effort to increase the patient's comfort and confidence during the assessment. Provide a warm place in which to change into a gown and a secure place to leave clothes and other possessions.

As you work through each assessment phase, tell the patient what is about to happen and mention if any of the procedures will be uncomfortable. Provide information about the results of the examination, when appropriate.

TOOLS OF THE TRADE

In addition to the basic tools described in Chapter 2, you will need an otoscope fitted with a nasal speculum and a magnifying lens. Chapter 2 contains information describing the use of these tools.

ASSESSMENT TECHNIQUES

When performing a respiratory examination, develop a sequential method of examination so that no areas are omitted and so findings can be compared accurately. It is especially important to note symmetry or lack of it. Be sure to compare, for example, the right apex of the lung to the left apex, not the right apex to the right base.

The examination should begin with an overall inspection of each area involved, followed by use of one or more of the following techniques: palpation, percussion, and auscultation.

NURSE ALERT:
In the infant and young child, breathing is generally diaphragmatic. Use of intercostal muscles and spinal extensor and neck muscles usually indicates dyspnea.

▲ Palpation

Palpation is described in Chapter 2. When used as part of respiratory assessment, it allows you to determine several important indicators.

Tenderness in any particular area can be explored through palpation. By gently palpating the patient's thorax, you can determine the range and radiation patterns of any tender areas.

An estimation of respiratory expansion can be made using palpation techniques. Place your hands on the patient's back, with the thumbs pushing toward the spine to raise a loose fold of skin. Tell the patient to take a breath, slightly deeper than usual. Your thumbs should move apart approximately 3 to 5 cm. Also note any asymmetry in movement when the patient inhales and exhales.

Tactile fremitus is also assessed via palpation. As you palpate the chest, have the patient repeat a short phrase, such as "ninety-nine" or "one-one-one." The vibration felt under the hand should be similar from left to right but is generally strongest at the apices and decreases approaching the bases. Decreased fremitus indicates air trapping, as with emphysema, and increased fremitus indicates a mass or fluid, as with a tumor or pneumonia.

▲ Percussion

General instruction in the technique of percussion appears in Chapter 2.

When using percussion in respiratory assessment, use indirect percussion, as shown in the illustration on the following page. As you move to new locations, the sound you hear will change. You must learn to distinguish slight differences in sound.

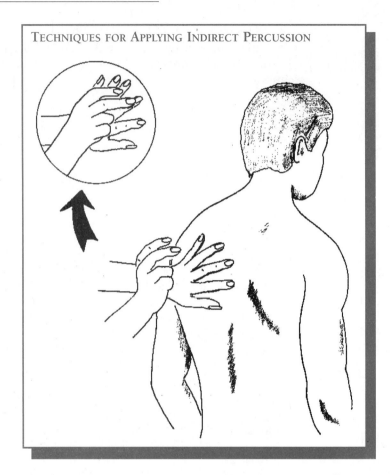

TECHNIQUES FOR APPLYING INDIRECT PERCUSSION

The five basic notes are resonance, hyperresonance, flatness, dullness, and tympany.

- Resonance is the normal note found in most healthy adults. This may be dulled slightly in either the obese patient or in the patient with a heavy muscular build.
- Hyperresonance may indicate overinflated lungs, sometimes an indication of emphysema or pneumothorax.
- Flatness or dullness may indicate fluid or solid tissue replacing normal air-filled lung space. This density may indicate conditions such as pneumonia, the presence of a tumor, or large pleural effusion.
- Tympany is an uncommon finding, which may be elicited when percussing over a large pneumothorax.

Diaphragmatic expansion can also be measured using percussion. Percuss along the scapular line as the patient inhales deeply and holds the breath. Note the point at which resonance changes to dullness. This marks the underlying change between resonant lung tissue and dull subdiaphragmatic tissue. Tell the patient to release the breath and exhale deeply. Percuss again and mark the change from resonance to dullness. The difference between these two points ranges from 3 to 6 cm, normally around 5 cm.

▲ Auscultation
General techniques for auscultation are described in Chapter 2. When using auscultation in respiratory assessment, listen for the normal sounds and patterns of the patient's ventilation and for any added, or adventitious, sounds.

NURSE ALERT:
When listening for breath sounds and patterns, especially during auscultation, be careful not to confuse ambient noise or the noise from equipment used to care for the patient with the actual sounds of ventilation.

Normal sounds are classified according to pitch and intensity and by the relationship of the inspiration phase to the expiration phase into three categories: bronchial, bronchovesicular, and vesicular.

• Bronchial sounds are normally heard in the area of the trachea and manubrium and are high-pitched and loud. The expiration phase lasts longer than inspiration and there is a brief pause between the two phases.
• Bronchovesicular sounds are medium in intensity and pitch and the inspiratory and expiratory phases are evenly matched. Sometimes you may hear a very brief pause between the two phases. These sounds can be heard in the first and second interspaces anteriorly and between the scapulae.
• Vesicular sounds are heard without a pause between the longer inspiratory phase and the shorter expiratory phase. They are soft, relatively low in intensity, and fade away during the expiratory phase. They are most easily heard directly over the lung.

▲ Adventitious Sounds
In addition to the normal sounds of breathing, as described above, you may hear additional sounds. These adventitious sounds fall into two broad categories: continuous and discontinuous or intermittent sounds.

- Continuous sounds include wheezes and rhonchi. Wheezes are created by air passing through airways obstructed by edema, tumor, or secretions. Rhonchi occur primarily during expiration and, like wheezes, are caused by air passing through narrowed airways. Wheezes are higher pitched than rhonchi and have a musical quality. The sound of rhonchi is more like snoring and it may vary with coughing.
- Discontinuous sounds include fine and coarse crackles and pleural rub. Crackles are caused by air passing through moisture or when air flows past passageways closed during expiration that open suddenly upon inspiration. Fine crackles are higher pitched, softer, and shorter in duration than coarse crackles. Pleural rubs are created when the inflamed pleural surfaces rub together. They sound like crackles but are located more superficially in the patient's chest.

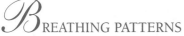

BREATHING PATTERNS

Breathing patterns are classified by rate, depth, and regularity. Normal adult respiration occurs at the rate of 12 to 20 breaths per minute, is quite even, and has a depth of 500 to 800 mL.

THE CHILD:
In children, the rate of respiration gradually decreases with age. A newborn's respiration rate is approximately 30 to 80 breaths per minute. By the age of two, this has dropped to approximately 20 to 40 breaths per minute. Teenagers and adults have respiration rates of 12 to 20 breaths per minute.

THE ELDERLY:
In the older patient, you may find a shallower breathing pattern. This is often due to the normal atrophy and loss of muscle strength that accompanies the aging process.

Changes in the rate, depth, or regularity of a patient's breathing pattern should be noted. Some of the more common abnormal patterns are:

- Tachypnea, in which the rate is faster, while the depth is shallower, but still even. This is a normal response to increased exertion, fear, or fever.
- Hyperventilation, in which the rate is faster and the depth is greater. The pattern is still even. It sometimes

occurs in response to extreme exertion, fear, or anxiety.
- Bradypnea, in which the rate is significantly slower than normal, but both the depth and the pattern remain normal. Bradypnea is often seen in comatose patients.
- Hypoventilation, in which the depth, pattern, and rate are irregular. This may be caused when the patient uses splinting to avoid pain on ventilation or it may be the result of an overdose of narcotic or anesthetic.
- Cheyne-Stokes respiration, in which rate and depth increase gradually and then decrease. This pattern is regularly interrupted by a period of apnea. This pattern is common during sleep in both children and older adults. It may also be seen in patients with severe congestive heart failure or terminally ill patients. It can be caused by uremia, narcotic overdose, and brain injury.
- Biot's respiration, in which the pattern is similar to Cheyne-Stokes respiration, except that the pattern of ventilation and apnea is irregular. It may be caused by brain injury or respiratory depression.
- Kussmaul breathing, which is deep breathing associated with metabolic acidosis. The respiratory rate may be fast, slow, or normal.

NURSE ALERT:
You may also see a pattern of normal breathing interrupted by sighing. Occasional sighs are normal; however, frequent sighing may signal emotional distress and may lead to hyperventilation.

RELATED DIAGNOSTIC PROCEDURES AND LABORATORY TESTS

Additional information to help in diagnosis can be found in the results of additional diagnostic procedures and tests.

The nurse plays a critical role in conducting many diagnostic tests and procedures. Assuring appropriate specimen collection, preparing for patient monitoring before and after invasive procedures, and educating the patient are all within the realm of the nurse's responsibilities.

Laboratory Tests

▲ Arterial Blood Gas (ABG) Analysis

ABG analysis measures four characteristics:
- the partial pressure of oxygen (PaO_2) and carbon dioxide ($PaCO_2$) dissolved in arterial blood plasma,
- the acid-base balance of the plasma,
- the amount of oxygen bound to hemoglobin, and
- the total content of oxygen carried in the blood.

At sea level in room temperature, the normal range of ABG levels are:
- PaO_2—80 to 100 millimeters of mercury (mm Hg)
- $PaCO_2$—35 to 45 mm Hg
- pH—7.35 to 7.45
- Bicarbonate (HCO_3)—22 to 26 mEq/L
- Oxygen saturation (SaO_2)—greater than 96%
- Oxygen content—18 to 20 mm/100 mL of blood (18% to 20%)

In interpreting blood gas values, decreased PaO_2 readings demonstrate hypoxemia or insufficient oxygenation of the blood. Increased $PaCO_2$ indicates hypercapnia, or an excess of carbon dioxide in the blood. $PaCO_2$ levels of 45 mm Hg or more indicate respiratory acidosis. Hypocapnia, or insufficient carbon dioxide in the blood, is indicated by low levels of $PaCO_2$. Partial pressure of carbon dioxide levels of 35 mm Hg or less indicate respiratory alkalosis.

In patients over 60 years of age, normal levels of PaO_2 are lower than these ratings. Levels of $PaCO_2$ do not change with age.

NURSE ALERT:
PaO_2 readings of less than 40 mm Hg indicate a life-threatening situation that requires immediate attention.

The HCO_3 level is a reflection of the kidneys' ability to maintain the acid-base balance in relation to changes in the body's respiratory and metabolic functions.

When evaluating oxygen saturation, consider the amount of available hemoglobin. Normal oxygen saturation with hemoglobin at 7 g is unable to deliver the same amount of oxygen as with hemoglobin at 14 g.

It's crucial to examine oxygen content in addition to the other indicators to determine oxygenation status. A change in PaO_2, oxygen saturation, and hemoglobin can influence oxygen content. A decrease in oxygen content can result in tissue hypoxia.

NURSE ALERT:
Arterial puncture sites must have firm pressure applied for approximately 5 minutes after the procedure and must be monitored for bleeding thereafter.

▲ Sputum Evaluation
Sputum evaluation is an important factor in many respiratory disorders. Sputum culture is used to determine if an infection is present in the respiratory tract. Specimens should always be collected in a sterile container to avoid contamination.

Sputum smear may reveal the same microorganisms as sputum culture but may also reveal eosinophils in the asthmatic patient, fungal organisms that may not appear in the culture, and other cells not normally seen in sputum. Therefore, it is important to complete both a culture and a smear test.

Sputum cytology examination is performed for determination of lung cancer. Malignant cells can be identified in approximately 50% of lung cancer cases via sputum evaluation.

▲ Throat Culture
Throat culture is used to identify infectious organisms in the throat when symptoms of pharyngitis or tonsillitis are present. Like the sputum culture, it must be collected in a sterile container, with a sterile swab. Bacterial, viral, and fungal organisms can be found via a throat culture.

▲ Skin Tests
The tuberculin skin test is used to detect infection with tuberculosis. The agent used is a protein fraction of the tubercle bacilli. When introduced into the skin of an individual with an active or a dormant tuberculsis infection, localized skin erythema and induration of the skin result. The method of choice for administering the test is by the Mantoux test, using a needle and syringe to give an intradermal injection. The injection site should be examined within 48 to 72 hours for evidence of a reaction.

Other skin tests for coccidioidomycosis or histoplasmosis are performed by an intradermal injection of antigens prepared from culture. Positive reactions appear within 24 to 72 hours. Erythema and induration of 5 mm or more indicate a positive reaction.

Diagnostic Procedures

▲ Pulmonary Angiography

Pulmonary angiography allows visualization of pulmonary vasculature by using injectable radiopaque dye. The dye is injected through a catheter threaded, by way of a peripheral artery, into the vessel to be studied. Thromboemboli, hemorrhage, trauma, tumor, and malformation of vessels causing obstruction of normal flow can be seen via this procedure.

As pulmonary angiography requires arterial puncture, the catheter site requires close observation during and after the procedure to prevent bleeding and compromise of neurovascular function.

NURSE ALERT:
Be aware of patient allergies. A history of allergy to iodine or dye should be noted.

▲ Computed Tomography (CT) Scan

CT is a diagnostic imaging technique that produces cross section pictures useful in identifying tumors, enlarged lymph nodes, infection, abnormal collection of fluid in body cavities, and infarction. It may be used in identifying, staging, and evaluating cancer and in evaluating pleural effusion and respiratory tract infection.

Intravenous contrast dye may be used to enhance the image; therefore, it is important to note any patient allergies to iodine or dye.

NURSE ALERT:
The equipment used for the CT scan requires that the patient be able to tolerate confinement in a small space and remain motionless for 30 to 90 minutes. Be sure to assess for a history of claustrophobia before sending the patient to this test. Also be sure that any pain the patient may be suffering is under control, as this may interfere with the patient's ability to tolerate the procedure.

▲ Magnetic Resonance Imaging (MRI)

Magnetic resonance imaging is a noninvasive diagnostic imaging technique that uses radio waves and a strong magnetic field to detect differences in the physiochemical components of the body. It is used to identify abnormalities in both the upper and the lower airway. There is no ionizing radiation involved in this procedure and it can often be completed without the use of contrast material. When contrast agents are needed, noniodine material is used and adverse reactions are rare.

NURSE ALERT:
Some MRI equipment also requires confinement and the ability to remain motionless for 30 to 90 minutes while the image is being created. Be sure your patient can tolerate these restrictions before scheduling the test.

▲ Radioisotope Scans

In radioisotope scans, radioisotopes are given intravenously to be absorbed by body tissue. Abnormal tissue, such as a tumor, generally absorbs more of the radioactive material than does normal tissue. In respiratory disorders, scans can detect pulmonary emboli, tumors, and perfusion changes.

▲ Pulmonary Function Tests

Pulmonary function tests are used to differentiate restrictive disorders from obstructive disorders and to quantify the severity of lung disease. These studies are frequently used at the time of diagnosis of lung disease to establish a baseline for comparison throughout the course of the illness.

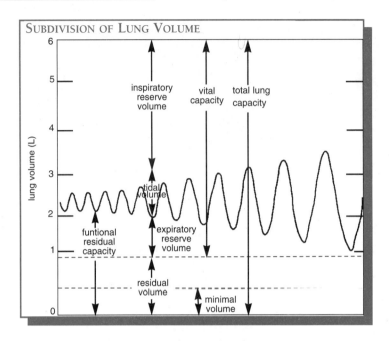

SUBDIVISION OF LUNG VOLUME

There are several pulmonary function tests:
- Tidal volume measures the amount of air inhaled and exhaled during quiet respiration.
- Inspiratory capacity measures the maximum amount of air inspired with one breath.
- Expiratory reserve volume measures the maximum amount of air that can be exhaled after a normal exhalation.
- Inspiratory reserve volume measures the maximum amount of air that can be inspired after normal inspiration.
- Vital capacity measures the maximum amount of air that can be exhaled after maximum inhalation.
- Residual volume measures the amount of air remaining in the lungs after maximum expiration.
- Functional residual capacity measures the amount of air remaining in the lungs after normal expiration.

▲ Chest X-ray

The chest X-ray is perhaps one of the most frequently used radiographic tests in evaluating lung disorders. It is useful in identifying pneumothorax, infection, effusion, adult respiratory distress syndrome, tumors and other masses, trauma, and pulmonary edema. Images are most commonly taken from three perspectives: posteroanterior, anteroposterior, and lateral.

▲ Bronchoscopy

Bronchoscopy is usually performed using a flexible fiber-optic bronchoscope to visualize the trachea and bronchi directly. In addition to visualizing these internal structures, the procedure can be used to obtain specimens and remove foreign objects and secretions.

The procedure is usually performed using some form of local anesthesia and sedatives. As with other invasive procedures, the patient must fast (NPO) for 6 to 8 hours prior to the procedure because of the risk of aspiration. Local anesthesia will also alter the gag, swallowing, and cough reflexes, so maintaining the patient NPO for 2 to 4 hours after the procedure is also critical.

Close monitoring of vital signs before, during, and after the procedure is critical to reduce the risk of complications, such as bleeding, pneumothorax, and airway obstruction.

▲ Laryngoscopy

Laryngoscopy is a procedure similar to bronchoscopy and allows direct visualization of the glottis, pharynx, and larynx. Because of its invasive nature and the use of local anesthesia and sedatives, monitoring as described for bronchoscopy is required for laryngoscopy as well.

▲ Thoracentesis

Thoracentesis may be performed for either diagnostic or therapeutic reasons. Under sterile conditions, a needle is inserted into the pleural space to extract fluid. If the specimen is needed for diagnosis, it is sent to the laboratory for culture and sensitivity tests and cytologic and chemical studies to determine its origin.

NURSE ALERT:
There is risk of pneumothorax and bleeding because of the nature of this procedure. Close monitoring of vital signs is required during and after the procedure.

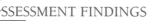

ASSESSMENT FINDINGS

Start the assessment with an overall examination of the patient for general signs of respiratory distress. Depending on the complaint bringing the patient to you (if there is one), examine the nose and throat or the chest and thorax.

ASSESSMENT FINDINGS

The information below describes general assessment techniques, followed by an examination of the chest and thorax and then an examination of the nose and throat. When assessing the chest and thorax, complete the sequence below for both the anterior and the posterior chest and thorax.

ASSESSMENT	NORMAL FINDINGS	DEVIATIONS FROM NORMAL
• Examine the patient for general signs of respiratory distress.	• Patient should be sitting comfortably with no obvious signs of pain or discomfort and breathing easily.	• Obvious signs of pain, including facial grimacing, splinting, shallow breathing, sweating, and flaring of nostrils when inhaling. • Signs of mental confusion or excessive drowsiness, which may indicate hypoxia.
• Observe for digital clubbing.	• Normal angulation of the nail is approximately 160 degrees. The nail root is secure and the curvature of the nail is not severe.	• Angulation of the nail is greater than 160 degrees and nail shows sign of extreme curvature. The nail root appears to float over the tip of the finger.

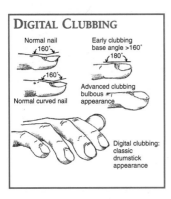

DIGITAL CLUBBING

Normal nail
160°

Early clubbing
base angle >160°
180°

160°
Normal curved nail

Advanced clubbing
bulbous
appearance

Digital clubbing:
classic
drumstick
appearance

ASSESSMENT FINDINGS (CONTINUED)

ASSESSMENT	NORMAL FINDINGS	DEVIATIONS FROM NORMAL
• Examine mucous membranes, lips, skin, and ears for signs of cyanosis or extreme pallor.	• These areas should be consistent with patient's overall skin color.	• Bluish tone to the skin or extremely pale skin.

TRANSCULTURAL CONSIDERATIONS
In dark-skinned individuals, the lips and gums may be bluish normally. Be careful not to mistake this for cyanosis. Careful inspection of the nailbeds, tongue, and buccal mucosa will usually reveal cyanosis. The conjunctiva may also reveal cyanosis.

In dark-skinned individuals displaying pallor, the skin may appear ashen-gray. In brown-skinned individuals, the skin may be yellow-brown.

ASSESSMENT FINDINGS (*CONTINUED*)

ASSESSMENT	NORMAL FINDINGS	DEVIATIONS FROM NORMAL
• Inspect the nose, lips, mouth, and tongue for color, shape, contour, and lesions.	• Normal skin is consistent with the patient's overall coloring. • Formation of the nose is symmetric. Breathing is easy, with no evidence of nasal flaring. The tongue is pinkish red and has a roughened surface. • All areas are free of lesions or inflammation. **THE ELDERLY:** In the older patient, you may see drier and paler mucous membranes.	• Signs of cyanosis or extreme pallor. • Signs of respiratory difficulty, such as nasal flaring and intercostal retraction. • Lesions or ulcerations. • Extremely red or swollen tongue. • Extreme dryness or excessive amounts of saliva. • Gums that bleed easily.

ASSESSMENT FINDINGS (CONTINUED)

ASSESSMENT	NORMAL FINDINGS	DEVIATIONS FROM NORMAL
• Using the nasal speculum or oto-scope, if a nasal speculum is not available, inspect the nasal area, noting the presence of foreign objects, lesions, bleeding, deviated septum, or perforations in the septum.	• Normal nasal tissue is reddish and moist. • The turbinates are similarly red in color. **NURSE ALERT:** Be especially careful when inspecting the turbinates. They are very tender and may bleed easily if scratched by the speculum.	• Signs of bleeding or presence of a foreign body. • Polyps or other growths. • Discharge or swollen, pale, or gray mucosa. • Formation that looks like a shelf in one nostril may indicate a deviated septum. • A perforated septum is indicated when the light shone in one nostril appears in the other nostril. • Septal perforation may indicate trauma or use of intranasal cocaine.

ASSESSMENT FINDINGS (CONTINUED)

ASSESSMENT	NORMAL FINDINGS	DEVIATIONS FROM NORMAL
• Using the tongue depressor, inspect the throat, tonsils, and uvula. Instruct the patient to say "Ah."	• Intact tissue is pinkish red, like the mouth. • Tonsils should be the same pinkish color. • The uvula and soft palate rise as the patient speaks. **T** **TRANSCULTURAL CONSIDERATIONS:** You may see a bifid uvula, which is a split uvula. This is common in Asians and native Americans, but rare in whites and blacks.	• Erythema, pallor, or evidence of cyanosis. • Edema or a whitish discharge covering the tonsils. • Strong breath odor such as a sweet fruity smell, the smell of ammonia or alcohol, or a foul odor, which may indicate infection.
• Inspect the patient's extended tongue.	• Patient should be able to extend the tongue evenly and with no difficulty.	• Tremors or pulling to the side as the tongue emerges from the mouth.
• Palpate the sinuses for areas of tenderness or pain.	• Patient should feel pressure but no pain.	• Evidence or expression of pain.
• Inspect the throat for symmetry and position.	• The trachea should be located at midline.	• Deviation from midline or any swelling or lumps.

ASSESSMENT FINDINGS (CONTINUED)

ASSESSMENT	NORMAL FINDINGS	DEVIATIONS FROM NORMAL
• Examine chest for lesions or scars, and note any iatrogenic devices in place.	• Skin should be lesion-free.	• Lesions such as petechiae, Osler nodes (reddish bumps on hands), erythema multiforme (red skin lesions).
• Examine chest for shape and configuration.	• Adult chest is symmetrical and wider than deep.	• Asymmetrical formations or signs that patient favors one side of the chest. • Abnormal conditions include barrel, funnel, or pigeon chest, as well as evidence of broken ribs. You may also see a deformity of the chest profile that is a result of spinal deformities.

THE ELDERLY:
In the elderly patient, you may see a smaller chest diameter. You may also encounter kyphoscoliosis, curvature of the spine, which may alter excursion.

ASSESSMENT FINDINGS (CONTINUED)

ASSESSMENT	NORMAL FINDINGS	DEVIATIONS FROM NORMAL
• Examine chest for shape and configuration. (continued)	**THE CHILD:** In the infant and young child, the chest is nearly round in shape, not wider than deep as in adults, and breathing is generally diaphragmatic. Use of intercostal muscles and spinal extensor and neck muscles usually indicates dyspnea.	
• Listen for normal breathing patterns, noting rate, depth, and regularity.	• Even ventilation, at approximately 12 to 20 breaths per minute.	• Abnormal breathing patterns such as hyperventilation, tachypnea, bradypnea, Cheyne-Stokes, or Biot's respiration. **THE CHILD:** In children, the respiratory rate is somewhat faster, from 30 to 80 breaths per minute in the newborn, to 20 to 40 in the 2-year-old, to the adult rate in teenagers. Any period of persistent or prolonged apnea may indicate an increased risk for sudden infant death syndrome.

ASSESSMENT FINDINGS (CONTINUED)

ASSESSMENT	NORMAL FINDINGS	DEVIATIONS FROM NORMAL
• Palpate for signs of tenderness or pain.	• Patient should tolerate palpation without discomfort.	• Indications or expressions of pain or crepitus, which is a crackling sensation felt under the skin. It may indicate subcutaneous emphysema, which is the presence of air in the subcutaneous tissue from a leak in the respiratory system.

NURSE ALERT:
Be especially careful during palpation if you suspect broken ribs. Deep palpation may shift bone fragments against internal organs.

• Palpate for tactile fremitus.	• Symmetrical sounds, stronger closer to throat.	• Decreased fremitus indicates an excess of air in the lungs, while increased fremitus may indicate a solid or fluid-filled area.

ASSESSMENT FINDINGS (*CONTINUED*)

ASSESSMENT	NORMAL FINDINGS	DEVIATIONS FROM NORMAL
• Measure approximate respiratory expansion.	• Chest expansion is between 3 and 5 cm.	• Decreased expansion may be the result of injury or pneumothorax. **THE ELDERLY:** In the elderly patient, you may see decreased respiratory expansion.
• Measure diaphragmatic expansion.	• Expansion of the diaphragm is 3 to 6 cm and is usually bilaterally equal. You may find a greater degree of expansion in the extremely athletic person.	• Large difference in symmetry during expansion or lack of significant expansion.
• Percuss the patient's chest wall to determine the probable composition of underlying tissue.	• Generally, you'll hear resonance over a normal air-filled lung and flatness over muscle. Percussion of the stomach yields a tympanic sound, while percussion over the heart yields a dull sound.	• Hyperresonance or normal sounds in abnormal locations.

ASSESSMENT FINDINGS (*CONTINUED*)

ASSESSMENT	NORMAL FINDINGS	DEVIATIONS FROM NORMAL
• Listen to the patient's breathing, using auscultation techniques.	• Vesicular sounds predominate; however, you may hear both bronchial and bronchovesicular sounds.	• Bronchial or bronchovesicular sounds in areas distant from the normal locations.
• Listen to the patient's voice when he or she is repeating a phrase such as "ninety-nine" or "one-on-one," followed by "e-e-e-e."	• Muffled sounds, indistinct words, and muffled "e-e-e" sound.	• Clear, loud speech (bronchophony) may indicate consolidated lung tissue. • The change of the "e-e-e" sound to an "a-a-a" sound (egophony) may also indicate consolidated lung tissue.
• Listen to the patient's voice as he or she whispers a repetitive phrase.	• Extremely muffled sounds, may be inaudible.	• Clear, loud speech (whispered pectoriloquy) may indicate consolidated lung tissue.
• Listen for any additional or adventitious sounds.	• No additional sounds should be heard.	• Continuous sounds, such as wheezes or rhonchi. • Discontinuous sounds, such as crackles or a pleural rub.

𝒮UGGESTED READINGS

Carpenter, K. D. "A Comprehensive Review of Cyanosis." *Critical Care Nurse* 13, no. 4 (1993): 66–72.

Grant, M. M., and M. B. McFarland. "Laboratory Tests of Acid Base Balance." *Nursing Implications of Laboratory Tests.* Albany, NY: Delmar Publishers, 1994.

Grossbach, I. "Case Studies in Pulse Oximetry Monitoring." *Critical Care Nurse* 13, no. 4 (1993): 63–65.

Guyton, A. C. *Human Physiology and Mechanisms of Disease.* Philadelphia: W. B. Saunders, 1992.

MacIntyre, N. R. "Respiratory Monitoring Without Machinery." *Respiratory Care* 35, no. 6 (1990): 546–556.

Misasi, R. S., and J. L. Keyes. "The Pathophysiology of Hypoxia." *Critical Care Nurse* 14, no. 4 (1994): 55–64.

Roberts, D. K., S. E. Thorne, and C. Pearson. "The Experience of Dyspnea in Late Stage Cancer." *Cancer Nursing* 16, no. 4 (1993): 310–320.

Szaflarski, N., and N. Cohen. "Use of Capnography in Critically Ill Adults." *Heart and Lung* 20, no. 4 (1991): 363–371.

SECTION III: CHRONIC OBSTRUCTIVE PULMONARY DISEASES

*C*hapter 7: Chronic Bronchitis

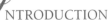

*I*NTRODUCTION

SEE TEXT PAGES

Chronic bronchitis is one of the pulmonary diseases generally called chronic obstructive pulmonary disease (COPD). It is often present in patients who also suffer from emphysema. Occasionally, patients suffering from bronchitis will also display symptoms of asthma.

Chronic bronchitis is characterized by excess production of mucus in the bronchi, causing chronic cough. To be considered chronic, these factors must be present for at least 3 months of the year for at least 2 years. The onset of the symptoms may be insidious and the patient may attribute many of them to the natural process of aging.

*S*UPPORTING ASSESSMENT DATA

If your assessment findings are similar to those listed here, they may suggest chronic bronchitis.

▲ Health History:
- Smoking
- Development of "morning" or "cigarette" cough
- Chronic, productive cough
- Dyspnea
- Exposure to industrial air pollution
- Presence of emphysema
- Frequent respiratory infections
- Family history of chronic bronchitis, or other chronic obstructive pulmonary disease
- Decreased ability to tolerate normal activity
- Aggravation of symptoms by dust, dampness, or cold

▲ Physical Findings:
- Purulent sputum
- Cyanosis
- Hypoxemia
- Hypercapnia
- Prolonged expiratory phase

- Rhonchi heard on expiration
- Tachycardia
- Abnormally high hemoglobin levels
- Cardiomegaly
- Low-lying diaphragm
- Edema
- Digital clubbing
- Increased bronchial thickening on X-ray

PATHOPHYSIOLOGY

The primary pathophysiologic feature of every COPD is an increased resistance to airflow, which develops over a long period of time. This resistance, in chronic bronchitis, is a result of increased mucus in the lungs and ineffective airway clearance.

The increase is a result of several factors. First, hypertrophy of the bronchial mucosal glands and an increase in the size and quantity of goblet cells cause an increase in the production of mucus. This is followed by a decrease in ciliated epithelium and impairment of the mucociliary clearance mechanism, leading to a decrease in the body's ability to rid itself of excess mucus.

As mucus collects in the lungs, stronger coughing is required to clear the airways. This stronger coughing damages the lung tissue. Pooled mucus provides an opportunity for bacterial and viral growth, leading to recurrent infection. In response to the infection, the lungs produce more mucus but are less able to clear the secretions.

The narrowing of the airways and the destruction of smaller bronchioles and alveoli may lead to a disruption in the gas exchange process, causing cyanosis, hypoxemia, and hypercapnia. Hypoxemia constricts pulmonary vessels, leading to pulmonary hypertension, as pressure in the right ventricle must increase to force blood into the constricted pulmonary vessels. The patient eventually experiences right-sided heart failure, also known as pulmonary heart disease or cor pulmonale.

*C*hapter 8: Emphysema

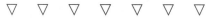

*I*NTRODUCTION

SEE TEXT PAGES

Emphysema is another of the pulmonary diseases generally called chronic obstructive pulmonary disease (COPD). It is often present in patients who also suffer from chronic bronchitis.

Emphysema is characterized by the loss of lung tissue elasticity and the abnormal enlargement of the alveolar ducts and alveoli, to the point of destruction of the alveolar walls. Because the lungs' capacity to adequately exchange gases is impaired, patients suffering from emphysema struggle to inhale more air.

*S*UPPORTING ASSESSMENT DATA

If your assessment findings are similar to those listed here, they may suggest emphysema.

▲ Health History:
- Family history of emphysema or other chronic obstructive pulmonary disease
- Smoking
- Exposure to industrial air pollution
- Presence of bronchitis
- Frequent respiratory infections
- Increasingly severe dyspnea without cough
- Decreased ability to tolerate normal levels of activity

▲ Physical Findings:
- Decreased breath sounds
- Weight loss
- Indications of breathing difficulty, including pursed lip exhalation and use of accessory muscles for inhalation
- Low-lying diaphragm with poor expansion
- Frequent hyperventilation
- Large lung capacity
- Large residual lung volume
- Prolonged expiratory phase
- Hyperresonance of the lung fields
- Normal heart size
- Decreased vascularity on chest X-ray or computed tomography scan

PATHOPHYSIOLOGY

There are two types of emphysema: centrilobular (the more common) and panlobular (also known as panacinar). The differentiation is based on the location initially affected by the disease.

Centrilobular emphysema involves first the respiratory bronchioles. Perforations develop in the bronchioles, more commonly in the upper portions of the lungs. As these perforations enlarge, a single air-filled space is created. Distal alveoli and alveolar ducts remain intact until the disease becomes more advanced.

Panlobular (or panacinar) emphysema is the less common type of emphysema and is characterized by the gradual destruction of the distal alveoli.

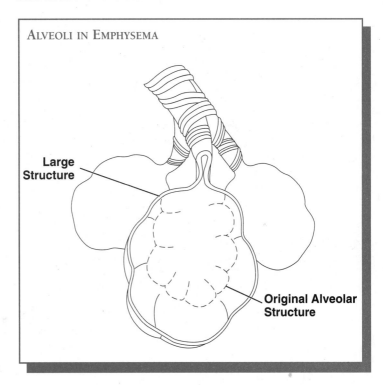

ALVEOLI IN EMPHYSEMA

Large Structure

Original Alveolar Structure

In either case, the capacity of the lungs to adequately complete gas exchange is impaired. As the disease progresses, the body responds to inflammation and infection by an increase in the alveolar microphages. These in turn destroy additional alveolar tissue, which continues to decrease the efficiency of the gas exchange process.

Chapter 9: Bronchiectasis

▽　▽　▽　▽　▽　▽　▽

INTRODUCTION

SEE TEXT PAGES

Bronchiectasis is a condition in which bronchial walls, weakened by damage to the mucosa and the muscle walls, become permanently dilated. Purulent secretions collect in the dilated areas. Chronic infection results, further weakening the bronchioles and perpetuating the condition.

SUPPORTING ASSESSMENT DATA

If your assessment findings are similar to those listed here, they may suggest bronchiectasis.

▲ Health History:

- Chronic, productive cough, often producing up to 1 cup of sputum a day
- Severe coughing spasms, especially when changing positions, as upon waking
- Dyspnea
- History of recurrent respiratory infections
- Overall weakness

▲ Physical Findings:

- Mucopurulent, malodorous sputum
- Hemoptysis (bloody streaks in sputum)
- Wheezes upon auscultation
- Fever
- Weight loss
- Anemia
- Digital clubbing
- Halitosis
- Bronchial wall thickening on chest X-ray, especially in lower lobes

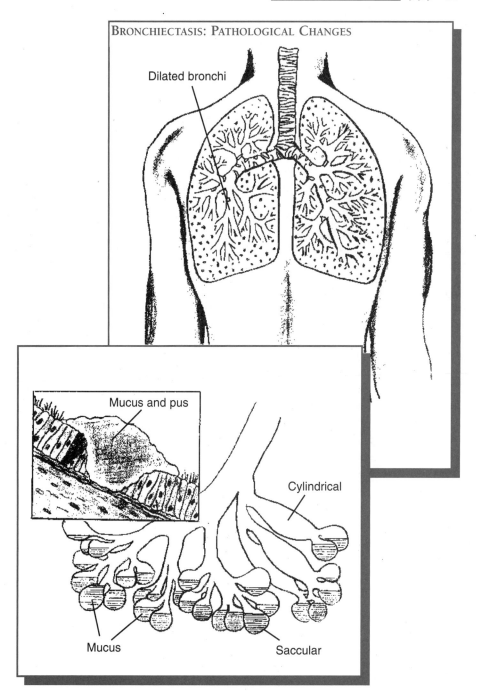

BRONCHIECTASIS: PATHOLOGICAL CHANGES

Dilated bronchi

Mucus and pus

Cylindrical

Mucus

Saccular

PATHOPHYSIOLOGY

Bronchiectasis develops as a result of the weakening of the bronchial wall. This weakening can occur with the aspiration of some foreign body, as a complication of such diseases as whooping cough, measles, cystic fibrosis, or influenza, or it can be associated with congenital respiratory defects. Once areas of the bronchial walls are weakened, they dilate, allowing purulent substances to settle in the cavities. The presence of the purulent material provides a medium for further infection, which weakens the bronchial walls even more. The continued obstruction causes areas of incomplete expansion and stretching of the bronchial walls, providing more cavities for the collection of purulent material.

$\mathscr{C}$hapter 10: Cystic Fibrosis

▽   ▽   ▽   ▽   ▽   ▽   ▽

$\mathscr{I}$NTRODUCTION

SEE TEXT PAGES

Cystic fibrosis is a hereditary condition in which mucus normally produced by the exocrine glands is abnormally viscid. It occurs in approximately 1 in 2,000 births. Although most cases are diagnosed during early childhood, 20% are diagnosed after age 15.

$\mathscr{S}$UPPORTING ASSESSMENT DATA

If your assessment findings are similar to those listed here, they may suggest cystic fibrosis.

▲ Health History:
• White
• Family history of cystic fibrosis
• Recurrent pulmonary infections
• Chronic pneumonia
• Decreased ability to tolerate normal levels of activity
• History of intestinal problems, including obstruction or diarrhea

▲ Physical Findings:
• Hyponatremia
• Hypochloremia
• Abnormally high salt content in sweat and saliva
• Increased chloride concentration in sweat
• Stunted growth in children and adults
• Bronchial thickening in the upper lobes on chest X-ray

In the older child or young adult, you may see classic signs of a chronic obstructive pulmonary disease (COPD): hypoxemia, cyanosis, purulent sputum, and tachycardia.

NURSE ALERT:
An indication of cystic fibrosis in infants is a salty taste when the infant's skin is kissed.

PATHOPHYSIOLOGY

Cystic fibrosis is characterized by an inability of chloride ions to cross the epithelial membranes of exocrine glands, causing increased viscosity and accumulation of mucus in the airways. Pancreatic dysfunction also occurs; causing steatorrhea (excessive fat in stool) and azotorrhea (excessive nitrogen in stool).

The highly viscid secretions that characterize cystic fibrosis cause obstructions in the bronchioles as well as in the pancreatic and hepatic ducts. Once the obstructions accumulate, airways become clogged and atelectasis may result. While approximately 85% of those with cystic fibrosis survive beyond 20 years of age, the most frequent cause of mortality is from COPD and related complications, such as cor pulmonale and respiratory failure.

*C*hapter 11: Asthma

▽   ▽   ▽   ▽   ▽   ▽   ▽

*I*NTRODUCTION

SEE TEXT PAGES

Asthma is one of the pulmonary diseases generally called chronic obstructive pulmonary disease (COPD). The primary pathophysiologic feature of every COPD is an increased resistance to airflow, which in asthma is a result of bronchospasm.

Asthma is additionally characterized by hypersensitivity of the tracheobronchial tree to various stimuli and is often associated with allergies. There are three types of asthma: extrinsic or allergic asthma, intrinsic or idiopathic asthma, and mixed asthma.

*S*UPPORTING ASSESSMENT DATA

If your assessment findings are similar to those listed here, they may suggest asthma.

▲ Health History:
• Occurrence of hay fever, eczema, or dermatitis
• Chronic bronchitis
• Prolonged attacks of dyspnea, sometimes followed by coughing that produces large amounts of whitish sputum
• Chest tightness
• Exposure to metabisulfites commonly used in food processing

▲ Physical Findings:
• Wheezing on auscultation
• Distant breath sounds, especially vesicular sounds
• Evidence of difficulty in expiration
• Profuse diaphoresis
• Tachycardia
• Tachypnea

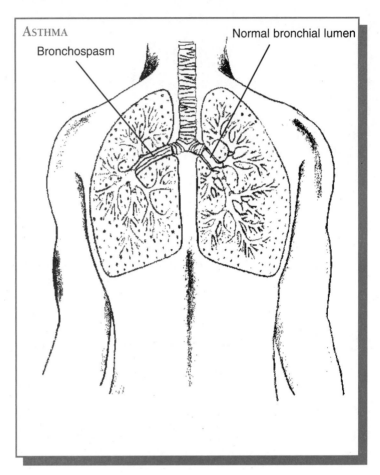

ASTHMA

Bronchospasm

Normal bronchial lumen

PATHOPHYSIOLOGY

Extrinsic asthma is found in a minority of adult asthma patients and is clearly caused by an allergen. Usually the allergen is in the form of an inhaled substance, primarily protein-based, such as animal dander. Occasionally, the allergy may be to a food such as milk.

NURSE ALERT:
Children suffering from extrinsic asthma often make a complete recovery by the time they reach adolescence.

Intrinsic asthma appears more commonly in adult patients, usually after the age of 40 and after the onset of infections of the tracheobronchial tree. It is more difficult to define a clear causative agent, but factors include colds, exercise, and emotional stress.

An asthma attack, in either extrinsic or intrinsic variations, follows the same pattern. Once the stimulus has sparked the attack, mucus production is increased and airways are constricted by bronchospasm and swelling of the mucosa. This combination results in air being trapped in the obstructed and narrowed passageways. This is reflected in the extreme effort the patient must make to expel air from the lungs. Uneven gas exchange occurs, which alters arterial blood gas values. It is possible that airflow can be restricted to such a severe degree that respiratory failure occurs.

SUGGESTED READINGS

Baker, K. L., and L. M. Coe. "Growing Up with a Chronic Condition: Transition to Young Adulthood for the Individual with Cystic Fibrosis." *Holistic Nursing Practice* 8, no. 1 (1993): 8–15.

Bone, R. C. "Chronic Obstructive Pulmonary Disease: Strategies for Detecting Disease and Slowing Progression." *Consultant* 31, no. 5 (1991): 21–27.

Janson-Bjerklie, S., S. Ferketich, P. Benner, and G. Becker. "Clinical Markers of Asthma Severity and Risk: Importance of Subjective as Well as Objective Factors." *Heart and Lung* 21, no. 3 (1992): 265–272.

Johannsen, J. M. "Chronic Obstructive Pulmonary Disease: Current Comprehensive Care for Emphysema and Bronchitis." *Nurse Practitioner: American Journal of Primary Health Care* 19, no. 1 (1994): 59–67.

Kee, J. L., and B. J. Paulanka. "Chronic Obstructive Pulmonary Diseases." *Fluids and Electrolytes with Clinical Applications*. Albany, NY: Delmar Publishers Inc. 612–618, 1994.

McKinney, B. "COPD and Depression: Treat Them Both." *RN* 57, no. 4 (1994): 48–50.

Schaffer, S. D. "Current Approaches in Adult Asthma: Assessment, Education and Emergency Management." *Nurse Practitioner* 16, no. 12 (1990): 18, 20, 23.

Stockdale-Wooley, R. "Overview of Lung Disease: Screening and Prevention." *Nurse Practitioner Forum* 4, no. 1 (1993): 11–15.

Tomezsko, J. L., T. F. Scanlin, and V. A. Stallings. "Body Composition of Children with Cystic Fibrosis with Mild Clinical Manifestations Compared with Normal Children." *American Journal of Clinical Nutrition* 59, no. 1 (1994): 123–128.

Wanner, A. "The Role of Mucus in Chronic Obstructive Pulmonary Disease." *Chest: The Cardiopulmonary Journal* 97, no. 2 (1990): Supplement 11S–15S.

Webb, A. K., and T. J. David. "Clinical Management of Children and Adults with Cystic Fibrosis." *British Medical Journal* (February 12, 1994): 459–462.

Whitney, L. "Chronic Bronchitis and Emphysema: Airing the Differences." *Nursing* 22, no. 3 (1992): 34–42.

Chapter 12: Tonsillitis, Pharyngitis, and Epiglottiditis

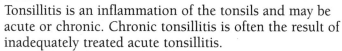

INTRODUCTION

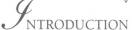

SEE TEXT PAGES

Tonsillitis is an inflammation of the tonsils and may be acute or chronic. Chronic tonsillitis is often the result of inadequately treated acute tonsillitis.

Pharyngitis, or acute sore throat, is almost always caused by infection. Occasionally, you may find that pain, when accompanied by inflammation or ulceration of the pharyngeal tissue, is caused by exposure to radiation or chemicals.

Epiglottiditis or supraglottiditis is an acute inflammation of the epiglottis and surrounding tissue. Typically seen in children, it may occur in adults as well. Rapid onset of inflammation and edema may result in airway obstruction, so prompt recognition and treatment are imperative.

SUPPORTING ASSESSMENT DATA: TONSILLITIS

If your assessment findings are similar to those listed here, they may suggest tonsillitis.

▲ **Health History:**
• Chills
• Earache
• Sore throat
• Pain on swallowing
• Constant desire to swallow
• General malaise
• Muscle and joint pain
• Extreme bad breath

▲ Physical Findings:
- Fever
- Tender lymph nodes
- Foul-smelling white or yellow exudate on tonsils
- Swollen tonsils
- Grayish tongue coating

𝒫ATHOPHYSIOLOGY

Acute tonsillitis is frequently the result of infection by beta-hemolytic streptococci and is more commonly found in children. Chronic tonsillitis is often the result of inadequately treated acute tonsillitis, although in adults, anaerobic bacteria may also be implicated.

At times, peritonsillar abscesses may form as a complication of acute tonsillitis. Symptoms and physical findings of tonsillitis are intensified in the presence of these abscesses as well as nausea, dehydration, trismus, and localized or systemic sepsis.

𝒮UPPORTING ASSESSMENT DATA: PHARYNGITIS

If your assessment findings are similar to those listed here, they may suggest pharyngitis.

▲ Health History:
- Pain on swallowing
- Scratchy or sore throat
- General malaise
- Headache
- Sensation of a lump in the throat

▲ Physical Findings:
- Inflammation of pharyngeal wall
- Generalized erythema of pharyngeal tissue
- Mild fever
- White exudate
- Shallow ulcers in pharynx

𝒫ATHOPHYSIOLOGY

Pharyngitis may be acute or chronic and may be caused by viral or bacterial agents, the growth of neoplasms, or irritation from chemical or environmental substances. Bacterial pharyngitis is more common in children and is usually caused by beta-hemolytic streptococci, while viral pharyngitis is more common in adults and may accompany the common cold or other inflammations of the upper respiratory tract.

Streptococcal infection causes the production of the pus commonly associated with pharyngitis. This provides a medium for further spread of the streptococci. These organisms also produce toxins that cause injury to blood cells and cardiac tissue.

Viral infection invokes the body's immune response and stimulates the collection of immunocompetent cells at the site of infection. These cells, in performing their function, lead to the inflammation and irritation associated with pharyngitis.

Chronic pharyngitis is caused by direct irritation of the pharyngeal tissues. This irritation may be the result of smoking or the inhalation of dust or other allergens. It may accompany chronic sinusitis or chronic dry mouth.

SUPPORTING ASSESSMENT DATA: EPIGLOTTIDITIS

If your assessment findings are similar to those listed here, they may suggest epiglottiditis.

▲ Health History:
- Sore throat
- Recent upper respiratory tract infection
- Dysphagia
- Restlessness
- Dyspnea

▲ Physical Findings:
- Fever
- Tachycardia
- Hypoxia/hypercapnia as indicated by arterial blood gas values
- Muffled voice
- Large, bright red epiglottis on inspection
- Drooling
- Mouth breathing with hyperextension of the neck

NURSE ALERT:
Stridor, severe dyspnea, nasal flaring, and use of accessory muscles signal impending airway obstruction.

PATHOPHYSIOLOGY

The most common infectious agent in epiglottiditis is *Haemophilius influenzae,* but infection may also be caused by group A streptococcus or pneumococci. Rapidly progressive inflammation and edema lead to difficulty swallowing even oral secretions. The voice is muffled rather than hoarse because the area affected is above the larynx. To identify the organism, both throat cultures and blood cultures may be done.

Diagnosis may be made by direct laryngoscopy. However, this procedure should not be done without appropriate personnel and equipment needed to perform endotracheal intubation or tracheostomy.

THE CHILD:

In the pediatric patient, it is important to distinguish between epiglottiditis and croup (acute laryngotracheobronchitis). While both may cause obstruction and acute inflammation, the causal agents and treatments vary.

*C*hapter 13: Sinusitis

▽   ▽   ▽   ▽   ▽   ▽   ▽

*I*NTRODUCTION

SEE TEXT PAGES

Sinusitis is inflammation of the sinuses and can be classified as either acute or chronic. Frequently, the patient suffering from acute sinusitis will have recently suffered a
viral upper respiratory tract infection. The chronic sinusitis
sufferer may find the symptoms occur in response to allergies or because of some physical defect, such as a deviated
septum.

*S*UPPORTING ASSESSMENT DATA

If your assessment findings are similar to those listed here,
they may suggest sinusitis.

▲ Health History:
- Nasal congestion, especially in the morning
- Pain or pressure in affected sinus
- Fatigue
- General malaise
- Decreased sense of smell
- Sensation of fullness or stuffiness in the head
- Headache, which may worsen with bending over or lying
  down
- Cough
- Sore throat
- Laryngitis

NURSE ALERT:
Often the patient will describe the symptoms as "a cold
that just won't go away."

▲ Physical Findings:
- Fever
- Facial pain or tenderness on palpation of the sinuses
- Purulent nasal discharge, usually yellow
- Limited transillumination because of the presence of
  purulent substances

*P*ATHOPHYSIOLOGY

Organisms causing the common cold are the most frequent
cause of acute sinusitis. The sinuses become blocked with
excessive mucus and this provides an environment for bacterial growth.

In chronic sinusitis, the infection is long-standing and does permanent damage to the epithelium. Once damaged in this way, the normal ciliary clearance mechanism operates less efficiently, causing a vicious cycle of recurrent infection and further damage.

*S*UGGESTED READINGS

Ahlers, L. K. "Recognizing and Treating Sinusitis in Children." *Physician Assistant* 14, no. 1 (1990): 35–37.

Carter, S. P. "Upper Respiratory Infections: The Common Cold and Its Complications." *Physician Assistant* 15, no. 12 (1991): 16, 18–20, 29–32.

"Sinusitis and HIV Infection." *Emergency Medicine* 25, no. 10 (1993): 46, 48.

𝒞hapter 14: Pneumonia

▽ ▽ ▽ ▽ ▽ ▽ ▽

𝓘NTRODUCTION

SEE TEXT PAGES

Pneumonia is a common respiratory disease and is a severe inflammation of the pulmonary tissue. There are several types of pneumonia, classified according to the affected areas of the lung. Bronchopneumonia involves patchy areas in several lobules of the lung. Interstitial pneumonia affects the wall around the bronchioles and alveoli. Lobar pneumonia affects a large portion of a lobe.

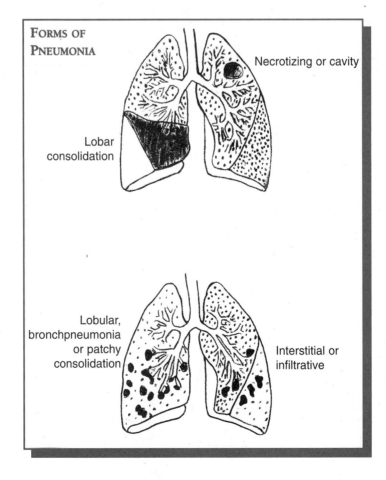

FORMS OF
PNEUMONIA

Necrotizing or cavity

Lobar
consolidation

Lobular,
bronchpneumonia
or patchy
consolidation

Interstitial or
infiltrative

PNEUMONIA CHARACTERISTICS AND TYPES

CHARACTERISTICS	TYPE: BACTERIAL	
	Pneumococcal	Staphylococcal
Temperature	Sustained fever 102°–106°	Sustained or intermittent fever 102°–105°
Respiratory Pattern	Shallow, rapid	Rapid
Adventitious Sounds	Pleural rub	Variable
Chills	Yes, shaking at onset	Yes
Pleural Pain	Yes	Yes
Sputum	Rust-colored	Hemoptysis purulent
Cough	Productive	Productive
Dyspnea	Yes	Yes
Cyanosis	Yes	Yes
Infecting Agent	*Streptococcus pneumoniae*	*Staphylococcus aureus*
Other Findings	Diaphoresis Nasal flaring Tachycardia General malaise	

TYPE: BACTERIAL *(CONTINUED)*

Klebsiella	Legionella	Pseudomonas
Remittent fever 102°–105°	Sustained fever 102°–105°	Reversal of diurnal temperature curve
Shallow, grunting	Shallow	Rapid
Crackles	Crackles	Diffuse crackles
Yes	Yes	Yes
Yes, severe	No	Yes
Thick, red nonpurulent (currant jelly)	Scant, purulent	Copious, yellow or green
Productive	Dry, nonprodutive	Severe
Yes	Yes	Yes
Yes	Variable	Variable
Klebsiella pneumoniae	*Legionella*	*Pseudomonas*
Common in alcoholics and diabetics	Common in elderly men who may also present with diarrhea, delirium, and abdominal pain	

PNEUMONIA CHARACTERISTICS AND TYPES (*CONTINUED*)

CHARACTERISTICS	TYPE: OTHER	
	Pneumocystis Carinii	**Viral**
Temperature	No	Fever
Respiratory Pattern	Shallow, rapid	Variable
Adventitious Sounds	Crackles (possibly)	Crackles
Chills	Yes	Yes
Pleural Pain	No	Variable
Sputum	Clear or white	Scant, may be bloody
Cough	Nonproductive	Dry, nonproductive
Dyspnea	Yes	Yes
Cyanosis	Yes	Variable
Infecting Agent	*Pneumocystis carinii*	Assorted viral agents
Other findings	Both PCP and fungal pneumonia often accompany HIV infection or immunosuppressive therapy (steroid therapy or organ transplant recipients).	

GRAM-NEGATIVE VARIATIONS

Fungal	Aspiration
Variable	Sustained
Rapid	Rapid
Variable	Crackles
Rare	Possibly
Yes, poorly localized	Yes
Scant	Foul smelling
Nonproductive	Productive
Yes	Yes
No	Variable
Histoplasma capsulatum, Coccidioides- immitis, Crytococcus neoformans, Aspergillus fumigatus	
	Uncommon in healthy individ- uals

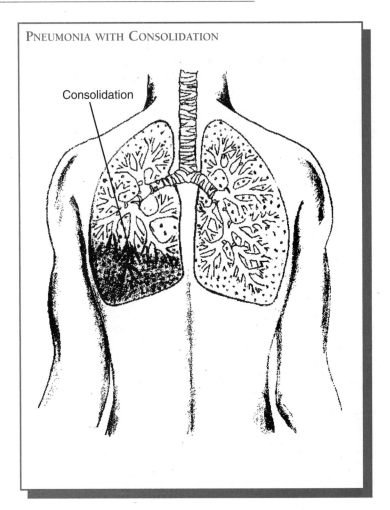

Pneumonia with Consolidation

Consolidation

℘ATHOPHYSIOLOGY

Once infection has occurred, usually from the inhalation of the infectious agent, different areas of the lung are affected. This depends on the infecting agent, the strength of the patient's immune system, and the presence of additional risk factors.

Infection causes damage to the lung tissue, reducing its ability to cleanse itself of mucus and reducing its elasticity. The resulting collection of material in the lungs provides an ideal growth medium for continued infection. Additional factors that worsen the condition include damage to alveolar tissue by cigarette smoke, malnutrition, or chronic infection; immunosuppression; and suppression or absence of the cough reflex.

Untreated, the infection can spread to the lymph system and from there to the bloodstream, causing systemic sepsis. In individuals with chronic lung disease, even mild infection can rapidly lead to respiratory failure. Early assessment and treatment are essential.

Aspiration pneumonia may occur in two forms: aspiration of gastric contents, which causes chemical injury to bronchial mucosa, and leads to fluid in the alveoli and destruction of surfactant, causing atelectasis; and aspiration of large amounts of grossly infected secretions from the upper airway, which causes necrotizing infection.

NURSE ALERT:
Pneumonia is more likely to cause death in patients with compromised immune systems, such as those patients with AIDS or cancer.

Chapter 15: Tuberculosis

▽ ▽ ▽ ▽ ▽ ▽ ▽

INTRODUCTION

SEE TEXT PAGES

Tuberculosis (TB) is an infectious disease caused by exposure to *Mycobacterium tuberculosis* via the respiratory tract, the gastrointestinal tract, or an open wound. Patients suffering from this disease will exhibit signs and symptoms of pneumonia and/or chronic bronchitis. Diagnosis of TB is confirmed when identification of *M. tuberculosis* is made.

SUPPORTING ASSESSMENT DATA

If your assessment findings are similar to those listed here, they may suggest TB.

▲ Health History:
- Fatigue
- Chest pain
- Dyspnea
- Alcoholism
- Malnutrition
- AIDS or other immunosuppressive conditions
- Ethnic background from countries where TB is prevalent
- Cough
- Night sweats
- Loss of appetite

▲ Physical Findings:
- Weight loss
- Rust-colored or blood-streaked sputum
- Positive TB test
- Evidence of calcified lung lesions in chest X-ray
- Fever, often greater than 102°F
- Acid-fast bacilli in sputum culture or smear

NURSE ALERT:
Symptoms of TB often mimic those of bronchitis or pneumonia. A TB test must yield positive results for a diagnosis
of TB. Alternately, there must be evidence of calcified
lesions shown via chest X-ray.

𝒫ATHOPHYSIOLOGY

Once the patient has been exposed to the mycobacterium
and tubercle bacilli are lodged in the alveoli, the pulmonary tissue becomes inflamed. Gradually the bacilli are
phagocytized and the alveoli become consolidated. This
process may result in the absorption of the bacillus so that
no residue remains or epithelioid cell tubercles are formed
by the microphages now present in the alveoli.

Necrosis of the tubercles takes two forms: caseous necrosis
or liquefaction. In the case of caseous necrosis, collagenous
scar tissue forms around the tubercle. In the case of liquefaction, the liquid material is sloughed into the tracheobronchial tree, resulting in small cavities. As these cavities
close, scar tissue is formed.

The formation of this scar tissue may block or restrict
bronchial lumen and may become the site of continued
inflammation. The disease is spread via the lymphatics and,
rarely, the blood vessels. When spread via the lymphatics,
the dissemination is slow and limited. When a blood vessel
is breached via necrosis of the nearby tissue, a large number of organisms can enter the bloodstream in a short time.

Chapter 16: Lung Abscess

▽ ▽ ▽ ▽ ▽ ▽ ▽

INTRODUCTION

SEE TEXT PAGES

Lung abscess is an infection of the lung parenchyma in which there is an accumulation of pus and the destruction of lung tissue. It is also called necrotizing pneumonia or pulmonary abscess. Patients suffering from chronic lung abscess may develop bronchiectasis.

SUPPORTING ASSESSMENT DATA

If your assessment findings are similar to those listed here, they may suggest lung abscess.

▲ Health History:
- Poor oral hygiene
- Gingivitis
- Productive cough
- Pleuritic chest pain
- Dyspnea
- Headache
- General malaise
- Chills
- Alcoholism

▲ Physical Findings:
- Foul-smelling purulent sputum, often brown
- Sweating
- Fever
- Weight loss
- Decreased breath sounds, pleural friction rub, or crackles on auscultation
- Dullness on percussion
- Empyema

*P*ATHOPHYSIOLOGY

Lung abscess may develop as a result of aspiration of nasal or oropharyngeal secretions. This often happens during periods of altered consciousness, such as anesthesia; during seizure disorders or periods of shock; or as a result of alcoholism. Sometimes the purulent material is caused by a periodontal condition.

If the infecting agent is anaerobic bacteria, the infection will be putrid. If the infecting agent is aerobic bacteria, the infection will be nonputrid. The abscess is accompanied by the accumulation of pus, which is the destruction of surrounding pulmonary tissue.

NURSE ALERT:
Lung abscess may also occur as a result of *Staphylococcus, Klebsiella, Proteus,* or *Pseudomonas* pneumonia.

*S*UGGESTED READINGS

Batt, M. D. "Update on Mycobacterial Issues for the Acquired Immune Deficiency Syndrome Era." *Journal of Intravenous Nursing* 17, no. 4 (1994): 217–219.

Chauhan, D. "Foul Smelling Sputum, Malaise and Night Sweats." *Respiratory Care* 37, no. 3 (1992): 273–274.

Couser, J. I., and J. Glassroth. "Tuberculosis: An Epidemic in Older Adults." *Clinics in Chest Medicine* 14, no. 3 (1993): 491–499.

Curry, J. L. "Identifying the Patient with Tuberculosis and Protecting the Emergency Department Staff." *Journal of Emergency Nursing* 20, no. 4 (1994): 293–304.

Elborn, J. S., and D. J. Shale. "Infections of the Airways." *Current Opinion in Infectious Diseases* 5, no. 2 (1992): 170–175.

Popa, V. "Airway Obstruction in Adults with Recurrent Respiratory Infections and IgG Deficiency." *Chest* 105, no. 4 (1994): 1066–1072.

"TB Increase Among Foreign-Born Changing American Epidemic." *TB Monitor* 1, no. 8 (1994): 110–111.

Timby, B. K. "Pneumocystosis in Patients with Acquired Immunodeficiency Syndrome." *Critical Care Nurse* 12, no. 7 (1992): 64–71.

SECTION VI: RESPIRATORY NEOPLASMS

𝒞hapter 17: Lung Cancer

▽   ▽   ▽   ▽   ▽   ▽   ▽

𝒥NTRODUCTION

SEE TEXT PAGES

Lung cancer, one of the most common cancers, is largely preventable. Generally, it is classified as small-cell lung cancer (SCLC) or non-small-cell lung cancer (non-SCLC). Non-SCLC is more common than SCLC.

𝒮UPPORTING ASSESSMENT DATA

If your assessment findings are similar to those listed here, they may suggest lung cancer.

▲ **Health History:**
• Age greater than 45
• Smoking
• Family history of lung cancer
• Exposure to environmental carcinogens, such as air pollution or asbestos
• Cough or a change in cough habits

▲ **Specific characteristics for SCLC:**
• Hoarseness
• Dyspnea
• Chest pain

▲ **Specific characteristics for non-SCLC:**
• Weakness
• Shoulder pain

NURSE ALERT:
Men who started smoking before age 15 and who have smoked one or more packs per day for more than 20 years are at greatest risk.

▲ Physical Findings:
- Weight loss
- Hemoptysis
- Digital clubbing
- Mass or effusion on chest X-ray

PATHOPHYSIOLOGY

Small-cell lung cancer is the rarer condition and is differentiated from non-SCLC by its poor prognosis, rapid growth rate, and brief duration of symptoms before diagnosis. Once present in the lungs, it spreads rapidly to the lymph nodes and submucosal vessels. Frequently, the tumors are located centrally, causing bronchial compression. Paraneoplastic syndromes, such as Cushing's syndrome and carcinoid syndrome, often accompany SCLC.

Further classifications of the more common non-SCLC include squamous cell carcinoma, adenocarcinoma, and large-cell carcinoma.

In squamous cell carcinoma, there is bronchial obstruction, ulceration, and bleeding. It generally occurs in central areas of the lung, especially where there is chronic damage to the epithelium.

Adenocarcinoma tumors are generally small and are found in areas of fibrosis and previous pulmonary damage. Vascular invasion is the most common route of metastasis.

The tumors of large-cell carcinoma are peripherally located and occur in any part of the lung. These large tumors quickly invade the nervous system and mediastinum.

Cancers of all categories affect the local lung tissue via airway obstruction, irritation, and inflammation. Tumors invade the mediastinum and pleural space. Patterns of metastasis vary based on the type of cancer and the severity of the disease when it is diagnosed.

$\mathscr{C}$hapter 18: Cancers of the Head and Neck

▽ ▽ ▽ ▽ ▽ ▽ ▽

$\mathscr{I}$NTRODUCTION

SEE TEXT PAGES

Cancers of the head and neck are primarily the result of the lifestyle and health habit choices an individual makes. Contributing factors include exposure to tobacco and smoke as well as to alcohol. These conditions include cancer of the oral cavity, oropharynx, larynx, hypopharynx, esophagus, nasal cavity, sinuses, nasopharynx, and salivary glands.

$\mathscr{P}$ATHOPHYSIOLOGY

Cancers of the head and neck generally originate on the surface of the mucosa. A number of etiological factors have been implicated in causing cancer of the upper airway. The inhalation or chewing of tobacco, the ingestion of ethyl alcohol, or a combination of the two is most frequently associated with cancer of the oral cavity, pharynx, and larynx.

Early cancers may appear white or red. As tumors increase in size, there may be local infection, necrosis, or bleeding. Typical tumors may be present as ulcerations or fungating masses or simply as roughening or thickening of the mucosa. With further tumor progression, there may be extension into the surrounding muscle, bone, or nerve tissue as well as blood or lymph vessels.

Although progression of the disease is generally local, there may also be metastasis to regional or distant sites via the lymphatic vessels and the venous circulation. The most frequent site of distant spread is the lungs, but there may also be metastasis to the bones, liver, and brain.

RISK FACTORS FOR CANCERS OF THE HEAD AND NECK

RISK FACTORS	ORAL CAVITY/ OROPHARYNX	LARYNX	HYPOPHARYNX
Sex	• Approximately 3:1 prevalence in men to women	• Higher in men	• Highest in men over 60
Smoking or other use of tobacco	• Yes	• Yes	• Yes
Use of alcohol	• Yes	• Yes	• Yes
Exposure to chemical irritants	• Yes, especially for workers in shoe manufacturing, asphalt, and cotton and wool industries	• Yes, especially for workers exposed to asbestos and for wood workers	• Not a contributing factor
Other	• Vitamin A deficiency • Poor nutrition • Poor oral hygiene	• Vitamin A deficiency • Vitamin C deficiency	• Incidence may be increased with vitamin B_{12} and iron deficiencies

NASAL CAVITY/ SINUSES	NASOPHARYNX	SALIVARY GLANDS
• Increasing nasal cancer in women • Increasing maxillary cancer in men	• Increased incidence in men, 2:1 over women	• Not a contributing factor
• Yes	• No	• No
• No	• No	• No
• Yes, especially to substances such as nickel, chromium, wood dust, shoe dust, hydrocarbons, and nitrosamines	**TRANSCULTURAL CONSIDERATIONS:** Chinese have a higher risk of nasopharyngeal cancer due to genetic predisposition and environmental factors, including high ingestion of salt-cured meat	• Exposure of head and neck to ionizing radiation

TRANSCULTURAL CONSIDERATIONS:
In Asian patients, you may find a history of chewing "pan" (a mixture of areca palm seed, shell, or slaked lime and tobacco) rather than a history of tobacco use through cigarette smoking or chewing tobacco.

SIGNS AND SYMPTOMS OF CANCERS OF THE HEAD AND NECK

SIGNS AND SYMPTOMS	ORAL CAVITY/ OROPHARYNX	LARYNX	HYPOPHARYNX
Pain	• Referred jaw/ear pain with oral cavity cancer • May experience local pain with oropharyngeal cancer but may be pain-free	• Throat pain with supraglottic involvement	• Throat pain or referred ear pain
Palpable masses	• Yes	• Yes, with glottic or subglottic involvement	• Cervical adenopathy
Other	• Painless color change in oral mucosa • Erythroplasia • Leukoplakia • Pigment changes • Sore throat • Dysphagia or odynophagia • Foul breath • Hemoptysis • Decreased function of cranial nerves V, IX, X, XII in advanced disease	• Dyspnea or stridor • Hoarseness, with glottic or subglottic involvement • Sore throat • Dysphagia or odynophagia	• Hoarseness if vocal cord invasion is present • Sore throat • Dysphagia or odynophagia • Absence of thyroid cartilage crepitus when moving laryngeal framework over cervical spine • Hemoptysis may be present • Weight loss

NASAL CAVITY / SINUSES	NASOPHARYNX	SALIVARY GLANDS
• Headache or facial pain	• No	• Ear pain
• No	• Cervical adenopathy, often painless	• Over glands
• Unilateral nasal obstruction • Asymmetry of the nasal cavity • Proptosis • Visual changes • Decreased sense of smell • Unexplained loosening of upper molars • Bony destruction • Nosebleeds • Incidence may be higher in those with chronic sinusitis	• Nasal obstruction • Bloody nasal discharge • Nasal quality to voice • Asymmetry of soft palate • Bulging or retracted tympanic membrane • Associated with Epstein-Barr viral infection • In advanced disease, findings include unilateral hearing loss, tongue paralysis, and trismus	• Facial palsy • Swelling of duct opening • Facial asymmetry

Chapter 19: Mesothelioma

▽　▽　▽　▽　▽　▽　▽

INTRODUCTION

SEE TEXT PAGES

Mesothelioma is an extremely aggressive tumor of the pleura, most frequently related to exposure to asbestos. In many cases, the exposure may have been brief or indirect. Wives of asbestos workers, for example, have an increased risk of mesothelioma. Onset of the disease occurs frequently many years after the asbestos exposure. Although once quite rare, its incidence is rising. Although they commonly occur in the pleura, mesotheliomas may also originate in the peritoneum, the pericardium, or, more rarely, the reproductive organs. Malignant pleural mesotheliomas are most commonly seen in men in their 60s and 70s. When the disease occurs in younger patients, it is usually associated with childhood asbestos exposure.

SUPPORTING ASSESSMENT DATA

If your assessment findings are similar to those listed here, they may suggest mesothelioma.

▲ Health History:
- Age greater than 50
- Male
- Exposure to asbestos
- Chest pain
- Dyspnea
- Cough

▲ Physical Findings:
- Bloody pleural effusion
- Weight loss
- Fever
- Pleural lesion on chest X-ray
- Digital clubbing
- Pericardial rubs

PATHOPHYSIOLOGY

Mesotheliomas occur most commonly in the pleura but may also appear in the pericardium and the peritoneum. The tumor invades the chest wall and then the lung, causing compression of the lung. It is a very aggressive cancer and metastasizes quickly into other areas by direct invasion. The area into which the cancer metastasizes depends on the primary site of the mesothelioma. Pleural mesothelioma often leads to metastasis in the lungs, brain, liver, lymph nodes, and adrenal glands. Abdominal mesothelioma often leads to metastasis in the pleura, lungs, pericardium, liver, and lymph nodes.

The cancer-causing effects of asbestos are probably a result of its physical properties. While most inhaled asbestos fibers are usually eliminated by coughing and other protective mechanisms of the respiratory tract, those that remain tend to lodge in the lower portion of the lungs near the visceral pleura. Inflammatory and fibrotic changes occur over a period of several years, which eventually promotes the growth of mesothelioma.

Dyspnea and nonpleuritic chest pain are common presenting symptoms and are frequently related to effusion. Tumors typically invade locally and involve thoracic structures, including the superior vena cava, vertebrae, ribs, esophagus, diaphragm, and spinal cord. Distant metastases are sometimes in distant lymph nodes, liver, brain, and adrenal glands.

SUGGESTED READINGS

Antman, K. H., H. I. Pass, T. DeLaney, F. P. Li, and J. Corson. "Benign and Malignant Mesothelioma." *In Cancer Principles and Practice of Oncology.* 4th ed. edited by V. T. DeVita, S. Hellman, and S. A. Rosenberg, 1489–1508. J. B. Lippincott: Philadelphia, 1993.

Craddock, C. "Head and Neck Cancer Prevention: The New Challenge." *Seminars in Oncology Nursing* 9, no. 3 (1993): 169–173.

Glover, J., and C. Miaskowski. "Small Cell Lung Cancer: Pathophysiologic Mechanisms and Nursing Implications." *Oncology Nursing Forum* 21, no. 1 (1994): 87–95.

Kusler, D. L., and B. A. Rambur. "Treatment of Radiation Induced Xerostomia: An Innovative Remedy." *Cancer Nursing* 15, no. 3 (1992): 191–195.

Lee-Chiong, T. L., and R. A. Mathay. "Lung Cancer in the Elderly Patient." *Clinics in Chest Medicine* 14, no. 3 (1993): 453–478.

Olson, J., and M. Frank-Stromberg. "Cancer Prevention and Detection in Ethnically Diverse Populations." *Seminars in Oncology Nursing* 9, no. 3 (1993): 198–209.

Potanovich, L. M. "Lung Cancer: Prevention and Detection Update." *Seminars in Oncology Nursing* 9, no. 3 (1993): 174–179.

SECTION VII: RESPIRATORY EMERGENCIES

*C*hapter 20: Pneumothorax and Hemothorax

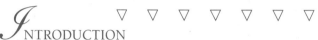

*I*NTRODUCTION

SEE TEXT PAGES

Between the covering of the lungs (the visceral pleura) and the lining of the thoracic cavity (the parietal pleura) is pleural space. This space is filled with between 10 and 20 mL of serous fluid, which serves to keep both surfaces in constant contact. This contact is a key component of the mechanism that keeps the lungs inflated.

Any substance entering the pleural space affects the lungs' ability to inflate properly. Pneumothorax is the accumulation of air in the pleural space and is frequently associated with trauma to the chest. Spontaneous pneumothorax may be related to chronic obstructive pulmonary disease (COPD) or other pulmonary disease. Iatrogenic pneumothorax may be created by several diagnostic and therapeutic procedures. Accumulation of blood in the pleural space is called hemothorax.

*S*UPPORTING ASSESSMENT DATA

If your assessment findings are similar to those listed here, they may suggest pneumothorax or hemothorax.

▲ **Health History:**
• Pleuritic chest pain
• Dyspnea
• Trauma to the chest

▲ Physical Findings:
- Fractured ribs
- Dislocated ribs
- Tachypnea
- Agitation
- Cyanosis
- No tactile fremitus on affected side
- Tachycardia
- Hypotension
- Decreased breath sounds
- No adventitious breath sounds
- Asymmetrical chest expansion
- Shift of trachea away from midline toward unaffected side
- Subcutaneous emphysema
- Collapsed lung shown on X-ray
- Hypoxemia
- Bulging of intercostal muscles on affected side
- Mediastinal emphysema
- High-pitched metallic sounds, synchronous with heartbeat
- Shock

Hemothorax only:
- Evidence of increased pleural fluid on X-ray
- Decreased hemoglobin and hematocrit

NURSE ALERT:
With pneumothorax, you may find hyperresonance on percussion, while with hemothorax, the finding will be dullness on percussion.

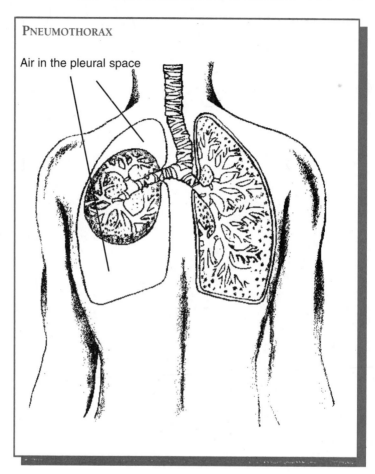

PNEUMOTHORAX

Air in the pleural space

PATHOPHYSIOLOGY

Pneumothorax is classified in several ways: primary, spontaneous, or simple pneumothorax; secondary or complicated pneumothorax; tension or trauma pneumothorax; and iatrogenic pneumothorax.

Primary or spontaneous pneumothorax occurs when subpleural air-filled blebs rupture, releasing air directly into the pleural space. The cause for the rupture of these structures in the absence of any pulmonary disease remains unknown.

Secondary pneumothorax occurs in conjunction with other underlying conditions, such as COPD. It may also be related to bronchiectasis, *Pneumocystis carinii* pneumonia, and

other diseases that weaken the alveolar walls and pleural
linings.

Tension or trauma pneumothorax occurs when an injury to
the chest or lungs allows air to penetrate the pleural space,
but not to escape it. Pressure rapidly increases within the
chest, causing displacement of the mediastinum to the
unaffected lung and impairment of blood flow. An open
pneumothorax or a sucking chest wound caused by trauma
is an opening between the pleural space and the open air.
Air moving in and out during respiration may cause a
sucking sound. A large opening may allow lung tissue to
prolapse.

NURSE ALERT:
Patients in cardiac arrest with pulseless electrical activity or
electromechanical dissociation may have pneumothorax.

Iatrogenic pneumothorax develops as a result of therapeutic or medical measures taken for other reasons. These
include anesthesia, central line placement, percutaneous
lung aspiration, and bronchoscopic forceps biopsy.

Hemothorax most often occurs as a result of chest trauma.
It may also occur as a result of thoracic surgery or pulmonary infarction.

NURSE ALERT:
In many cases, pneumothorax occurs with hemothorax.
This is referred to as hemopneumothorax.

*C*hapter 21: Chest Trauma

▽   ▽   ▽   ▽   ▽   ▽   ▽

*I*NTRODUCTION

SEE TEXT PAGES

Injuries to the chest are responsible for 25% of all trauma deaths in the United States. Chest injuries are grouped into two main categories: penetrating injuries and nonpenetrating or blunt injuries. In both cases, complications such as hemothorax, pneumothorax, shock, diaphragmatic rupture, and pulmonary contusion are common.

NURSE ALERT:
The patient's airway should always be assessed for blood, vomitus, or other secretions. In the unconscious trauma patient, the airway should always be protected.

*S*UPPORTING ASSESSMENT DATA

▼
▼
▼
▼
▼
▼

If your assessment findings are similar to those listed here, they may suggest trauma to the chest.

▲ Health History:
• Chest pain that worsens on inhalation and movement
• Dyspnea
• Recent injury to the chest (open or closed)

NURSE ALERT:
Blunt chest injury can result from motor vehicle accidents or falls from great height. Blows to the chest from steering wheels or blast injuries may create concussive forces causing injury to areas distant from the area of impact.

▲ Physical Findings:
• Bruised skin
• Pleuritic rub on auscultation
• Tracheal shift
• Tenderness on palpation
• Hypoxia
• Change in mental status
• Restlessness
• Paradoxical chest movements
• Cyanosis
• Tachycardia
• Hypotension

- Crepitus on auscultation
- Unequal chest expansion
- Hemoptysis

NURSE ALERT:
If the patient has suffered a ruptured diaphragm, you may also hear bowel sounds in the chest cavity.

ATHOPHYSIOLOGY

Penetrating injury to the chest is often accompanied by hemothorax and pneumothorax. It's most often caused by knife or gunshot wounds.

Blunt injury to the chest may take different forms: flail chest, pulmonary contusion, and diaphragmatic injury.

Flail chest occurs when one or more ribs are broken in at least two places. This creates a free-floating rib fragment, which may damage the underlying lungs. Generally, an indication of flail chest is that on inhalation, the uninjured side moves outward correctly, while the injured side moves inward. On exhalation, the uninjured side moves inward, while the injured side moves outward. The fragment poses great risk of injury to the internal organs.

Pulmonary contusion is damage to the structures of the lung so that the gas exchange process is interrupted. This includes bruising or hemorrhage of the interstitial or alveolar walls or alveolar collapse.

Injury to the diaphragm usually involves herniation of the muscle. It may accompany penetrating injury to the chest as well as blunt injury.

NURSE ALERT:
You may also see damage to blood vessels, especially shearing of the aorta and injury to the tracheobronchial tree when you encounter chest trauma.

$\mathscr{C}$hapter 22: Adult Respiratory Distress Syndrome

▽   ▽   ▽   ▽   ▽   ▽   ▽

$\mathscr{I}$NTRODUCTION

SEE TEXT PAGES

Adult respiratory distress syndrome (ARDS) is a type of respiratory failure that can be the result of many different conditions or diseases. It's not known why this syndrome presents identically despite the wide variety of causative factors.

This condition is also called shock lung, stiff lung, noncardiac pulmonary edema, wet lung, white lung, Da Nang lung, or adult hyaline membrane disease, although the term adult respiratory distress syndrome is the most widely accepted.

$\mathscr{S}$UPPORTING ASSESSMENT DATA

If your assessment findings are similar to those listed here, they may suggest ARDS.

▲ Health History:
- Dyspnea
- Orthopnea
- Mental sluggishness
- Trauma
- Sepsis
- Aspiration
- Smoke inhalation
- Drug overdose
- Surgery
- Shock

▲ Physical Findings:
- Hypoxemia, which cannot be relieved with oxygen administration
- Rhonchi on auscultation
- Tachycardia
- Tachypnea

- Extensive bilateral consolidation of lung on X-ray with normal heart size ᐧ

NURSE ALERT:
An early sign of ARDS may be diffuse, patchy infiltrates on chest X-ray.

PATHOPHYSIOLOGY

The alveolar-capillary membrane is normally permeable but only to the degree that it allows adequate gas exchange. With ARDS, this permeability increases, allowing the movement of red blood cells, white blood cells, and protein molecules into the interstitium and then the alveoli. A combination of inactivation of alveolar surfactant, decreased production of surfactant because the cells producing it are damaged, and the increased pressure in the interstitial spaces causes collapse of the alveoli. This, then, results in a lung that is stiff and difficult to inflate. Hypoxemia is the result of the decreased capacity for gas exchange caused by the collapse of some alveoli and the filling of others with fluid.

NURSE ALERT:
Common causes of ARDS include:
- Aspiration or inhalation injuries, such as
  - Near drowning
  - Aspiration of gastric contents or acids
  - Smoke inhalation
  - Inhalation of gases such as ammonia or phosgene
  - Prolonged inhalation of highly concentrated oxygen
- Infections such as
  - Pneumonia, both bacterial and viral
  - Tuberculosis
- Trauma such as
  - Head injury
  - Direct chest injury
  - Burns
  - Multiple fractures
  - Fat embolus
  - Multiple organ trauma

- Reaction to drugs such as
  - Heroin
  - Chlordiazepoxide
  - Methadone
  - Chloroform
  - Barbiturates
  - Colchicine
  - Propoxyphene
- Immune reactions
- Metabolic disorders
- Hematologic disorders
- Surgery
- Shock

Chapter 23: Acute Respiratory Failure

▽　▽　▽　▽　▽　▽　▽

INTRODUCTION

SEE TEXT PAGES

Respiratory failure occurs when the gas exchange process is no longer meeting the metabolic needs of the body. There are two forms of respiratory failure: type 1 or hypoxemic failure and type 2 or hypercapnic or hypoventilatory failure.

NURSE ALERT:
Several findings must be present for a clinical diagnosis of respiratory failure: extreme dyspnea, blood gas levels such that Pao_2 is less than 50 mm Hg breathing room air and $Paco_2$ is greater than 50 mm Hg, and respiratory acidosis as demonstrated by arterial pH measurements.

SUPPORTING ASSESSMENT DATA

If your assessment findings are similar to those listed here, they may suggest acute respiratory failure.

▲ **Health History:**
• Headache
• Mental confusion
• Tremors
• Slurred speech
• Anxiety

▲ **Physical Findings:**
• Tachycardia
• Hypertension
• Hypoxemia
• Hypercapnia

NURSE ALERT:
Some situations clearly indicate respiratory failure: someone is choking on food or is suffering cardiac arrest. However, when a patient suffers from some chronic respiratory conditions, respiratory failure can be a gradual and subtle change.

PATHOPHYSIOLOGY

In type 1 respiratory failure, you will see decreased oxygenation (hypoxemia) with normal or slightly lower levels of carbon dioxide. This usually occurs when there is a mismatch in the balance of ventilation and perfusion.

Adequate supply of blood to areas lacking ventilation results in perfusion without ventilation. Blockage of ventilation may be caused by adult respiratory distress syndrome, atelectasis, pneumonia, or pulmonary edema.

Decreased perfusion in areas that receive adequate oxygen supply results in ventilation without perfusion. Obstruction of blood flow is often the result of a pulmonary embolus or infarction.

In type 2 respiratory failure, you will see hypoxemia and increased levels of carbon dioxide (hypercapnia). This usually occurs because insufficient air is entering the lungs, and therefore, a smaller supply of oxygen is available for the gas exchange process. This may occur in areas where the air is thinner (high altitudes); where oxygen is being consumed by some other process, such as a fire; or where the oxygen in the area is being contaminated by another gas, such as carbon monoxide.

NURSE ALERT:
Respiratory failure can be caused by a number of diseases or conditions, such as:
- Depression of the respiratory center, related to drug overdose or head trauma
- Neuromuscular disorders, such as a cervical spine injury, amyotrophic lateral sclerosis, myasthenia gravis, or Guillain-Barré syndrome

- Pleural and chest wall injuries or disorders
- Chronic obstructive pulmonary disease (COPD)
- Pulmonary fibrosis
- Pulmonary edema
- Pulmonary embolism

In COPD, respiratory failure may be triggered by infections, allergic reactions with bronchospasm, trauma, heart failure, sedatives, anesthetics or narcotics, or changes in the viscosity or volume of tracheobronchial secretions.

*C*hapter 24: Pulmonary Edema

▽ ▽ ▽ ▽ ▽ ▽ ▽

*I*NTRODUCTION

The accumulation of fluid in the alveoli and interstitial spaces of the lung is called pulmonary edema. Increased resistance, which makes lung expansion difficult and interrupts the normal gas exchange, can rapidly pose a serious threat to the patient.

Pulmonary edema occurs as a result of increased microvascular pressure or increased permeability of pulmonary vessels to protein and solutes. This chapter addresses pulmonary edema related to cardiac disease.

*S*UPPORTING ASSESSMENT DATA

If your assessment findings are similar to those listed here, they may suggest pulmonary edema.

▲ Health History:
- Dyspnea, especially at night
- Orthopnea
- Productive cough
- Mental confusion
- Congestive heart failure

▲ Physical Findings:
- Tachycardia
- Tachypnea
- Crackles on auscultation
- Neck vein distention
- Cyanosis
- Copious, frothy, blood-tinged sputum
- Increased breath sounds
- Agitation
- Diaphoresis
- Elevated blood pressure

PATHOPHYSIOLOGY

Commonly, pulmonary edema is caused by left ventricular heart failure. The weakening or failure of the left side of the heart, combined with the continued functioning of the right side of the heart, results in an imbalance in pulmonary capillary pressure. This in turn results in the accumulation of fluid in the interstitial walls and then in the alveoli. As more and more fluid collects, gas exchange is impaired.

Chapter 25: Pulmonary Embolism

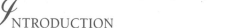

INTRODUCTION

SEE TEXT PAGES

The blockage of a main pulmonary artery or one of its branches by a blood clot, air, fat deposit, or other substance is called a pulmonary embolism. Depending on the size and location of the blockage, the condition may range from minor to life-threatening.

SUPPORTING ASSESSMENT DATA

If your assessment findings are similar to those listed here, they may suggest pulmonary embolism.

▲ Health History:
- Pregnancy
- Use of oral contraceptives
- Obesity
- History of heart failure
- Varicose veins
- Abdominal infections
- Cancer, especially pelvic masses
- History of deep vein thrombosis
- Sickle cell anemia
- Prolonged bed rest or long periods of travel in sitting position (such as on a plane or in a car)
- Dyspnea
- Apprehension
- Nausea
- Pleuritic chest pain
- Cough

▲ Physical Findings:

- Tachycardia
- Tachypnea
- Fever
- Cyanosis
- Diaphoresis
- Syncope
- Mental confusion
- Shock (almost always associated with massive embolism)
- Hemoptysis
- Pleural rub on auscultation
- Combination of wheezes and crackles on auscultation
- Reduced Pa_{O_2} on room air
- Evidence of decreased perfusion on isotope lung scan
- Petechiae over axillae and chest

PATHOPHYSIOLOGY

Embolic materials most often travel from distal sites to the lungs via venous circulation. When the embolus becomes lodged, an imbalance in the ventilation-perfusion ratio occurs. If there is complete obstruction, portions of the lung are not perfused, leading to infarction, which causes necrosis and hemorrhage.

SUGGESTED READINGS

Case, S. C., and C. E. Sabo. "Adult Respiratory Distress Syndrome: A Deadly Complication of Trauma." *Focus on Critical Care* 19, no. 2 (1992): 116–121.

Class, P. "Nursing Considerations for Airway Management in the PACU." *Current Reviews for Post-Anesthesia Care Nurses* 14, no. 1 (1992): 3–8.

Davis, L. A., and N. C. O'Rourke. "Pulmonary Embolism: Early Recognition and Management in the Post-Anesthesia Care Unit." *Journal of Post Anesthesia Nursing* 8, no. 5 (1993): 338–345.

Del Rossi, A. J. "Complications of Blunt Thoracic Trauma." *Trauma Quarterly* 6, no. 3 (1990): 65–74.

Guerci, A. D., and J. R. Michael. "Pulmonary Edema." In *The Principles and Practice of Medicine,* edited by A. M. Harvey, R. J. Johns, V. A. McKusick, A. H. Owens, and R. S. Ross. Norwalk, CT: Appleton and Lange, 1988.

Guinan, J. K. "Early Detection of Pulmonary Embolism." *Rehabilitation Nursing* 17, no. 4 (1992): 199–201.

Luchtefeld, W. B. "Pulmonary Contusion." *Focus on Critical Care* 17, no. 6 (1990): 482–488.

Papadakos, P. J., D. S. Johnson, et al. "Adult Respiratory Distress Syndrome: A Consideration with Rapid Respiratory Decompensation in Association with Preeclampsia." *American Journal of Critical Care* 2, no. 1 (1993): 65–67.

Reed, L. J., and M. J. Keegan. "Fat Embolism Syndrome: A Complication of Trauma." *Critical Care Nurse* 13, no. 13 (1993): 33–38.

Sisson, M. C. "Amniotic Fluid Embolism." *Critical Care Nursing Clinics of North America* 4, no. 4 (1992): 667–673.

Sommers, M. S. "Potential for Injury: Trauma After Cardiopulmonary Resuscitation." *Heart and Lung* 20, no. 3 (1991): 287–293.

Stein, P. D., R. D. Hull, H. A. Salzman, and G. Pineo. "Strategies for Diagnosis of Patients with Suspected Acute Pulmonary Embolism." *Chest* 103, no. 5 (1993): 374–383.

Sue, D. Y. "Respiratory Failure." In *Current Critical Care Diagnosis and Treatment,* edited by F. S. Bongard and D. Y. Sue. Norwalk, CT: Appleton and Lange, 1994.

Thielen, J. B. "Air Emboli: A Potentially Lethal Complication of Central Venous Lines." *Focus on Critical Care* 17, no. 5 (1990): 374–383.

Witry, S. W. "Pulmonary Embolism in Pregnancy." *Journal of Perinatal and Neonatal Nursing* 6, no. 2 (1992): 1–11.

Chapter 26: Pleurisy

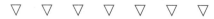

INTRODUCTION

SEE TEXT PAGES

Pleurisy is an inflammation of the visceral or parietal pleura. It can be caused by a variety of conditions or diseases and its most common presentation is that of sharp, unilateral pain of abrupt onset.

SUPPORTING ASSESSMENT DATA

If your assessment findings are similar to those listed here, they may suggest pleurisy.

▲ **Health History:**
• Pain that worsens with inspiration
• Dyspnea

▲ **Physical Findings:**
• Pleural friction rub on auscultation
• Coarse vibration on palpation
• Rapid respiration
• Splinting to reduce pain
• Decreased respiratory expansion
• Pleural effusion on X-ray

PATHOPHYSIOLOGY

The pain associated with pleurisy is caused by an inflammation of the nerve endings found in the parietal pleura. The visceral pleura does not contain nerve endings. As ventilation occurs and the two surfaces slide against each other, the pain increases as the nerve endings are stimulated.

NURSE ALERT:
Pleurisy can be the result of many other diseases and conditions, such as:
- Pulmonary infections, such as pneumonia and tuberculosis
- Viral infection
- Rheumatic diseases, such as systemic lupus erythematosus and rheumatoid arthritis
- Pulmonary infarction
- Chest trauma
- Cancer
- Autoimmune pleuropericardial inflammation after myocardial infarction (Dressler's syndrome)
- Uremia

Inquire about these diseases and conditions when taking the history of a patient with suspected pleurisy.

$\mathscr{C}$hapter 27: Pleural Effusion

▽ ▽ ▽ ▽ ▽ ▽ ▽

$\mathscr{I}$NTRODUCTION

SEE TEXT PAGES

Collection of fluid in the pleural space is pleural effusion. This space normally contains a small amount of serous fluid, which serves to keep the parietal and visceral pleuras in constant contact. The movement of blood, transudate, exudate, or chyle into this space occurs when the rate at which material enters the space is greater than the rate at which material is removed from the space.

$\mathscr{S}$UPPORTING ASSESSMENT DATA

If your assessment findings are similar to those listed here, they may suggest pleural effusion.

▲ Health History:
- Chest pain, if inflammation is also present
- Dyspnea, if large volumes of fluid are present
- Congestive heart failure
- Pulmonary infection
- Chest trauma
- Rheumatic disease
- Liver disease with ascites
- Cancer, primary lung or metastatic

▲ Physical Findings:
- Mediastinal shift away from affected side, if effusion is large
- Dullness or flatness on percussion
- Decreased or absent breath sounds
- Bronchial breathing or egophony over adjacent lung
- Evidence of fluid accumulation on X-ray with lung compressed over large effusion

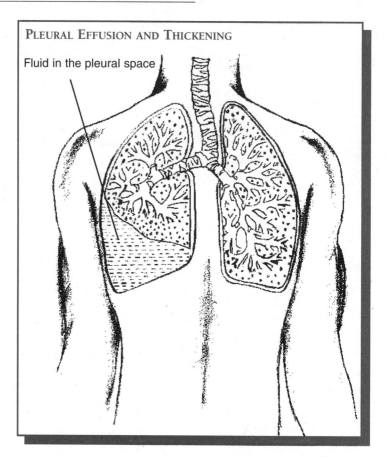

PLEURAL EFFUSION AND THICKENING

Fluid in the pleural space

𝒫ATHOPHYSIOLOGY

Deficiencies in any of the different functions of the lung can cause development of pleural effusion. These deficiencies may be caused by a variety of diseases and conditions resulting in changes in the capillary pressure, colloidal osmotic pressure, or intrapleural pressure; inefficient lymph drainage; and increased permeability of the capillary membrane.

Protein content of the material invading the pleural space determines whether it is a transudate or an exudate. Transudative effusions are caused by elevated systemic or pulmonary venous pressure or decreased oncotic pressure. Exudative effusions are from inflammation or other conditions of the pleural surface or lymphatic obstruction. If the material has a protein content of less than 3 g/mL, it's transudate; a protein content over 3 g/mL indicates an exudate.

Chylothorax, or accumulation of lymph, is caused by an interruption of the thoracic duct, which can be the result of injury, inflammation, or cancer.

Bleeding into the pleural space can be caused by trauma, as a consequence of chest surgery, the rupture of a blood vessel within the thoracic cavity, or cancer.

Hydrothorax, or the presence of increased levels of the serous fluid normally found in the pleural space, is most commonly a result of congestive heart failure.

$\mathscr{C}$hapter 28: Pulmonary Fibrosis

▽   ▽   ▽   ▽   ▽   ▽   ▽

$\mathscr{I}$NTRODUCTION

SEE TEXT PAGES

Pulmonary fibrosis is a general term for a collection of diseases whose effect on the lungs is that of restriction. Generally, the lung parenchyma stiffens, making respiration an ongoing struggle. Although the causes of these fibrotic changes vary from occupational diseases such as black lung, to diseases caused by exposure to toxic substances, to diseases with unknown origins, patients exhibit the same symptoms.

$\mathscr{S}$UPPORTING ASSESSMENT DATA

If your assessment findings are similar to those listed here, they may suggest a disease in the general class of pulmonary fibrosis.

▲ Health History:
- Dyspnea, which may be abrupt in onset
- Nonproductive cough
- Exposure to asbestos or other industrial pollutants, such as beryllium, coal, talc, and organic dusts
- Exposure to chemotherapeutic agents, including nitrosoureas, alkylating agents, and bleomycin
- Radiation exposure
- Decreased tolerance for exercise or exertion
- Sarcoidosis
- Scleroderma
- Chronic pneumonia or other lung infections
- Chronic pulmonary edema

▲ Physical Findings:

- Tachypnea
- Digital clubbing
- Reduced vital capacity, total lung capacity, and residual volume in pulmonary function tests
- Reduced arterial PaO_2 with low $PaCO_2$
- Fever
- Linear shadows or gross shrinkage or distortion of lung parenchyma on X-ray

PULMONARY FIBROSIS—DIFFUSE

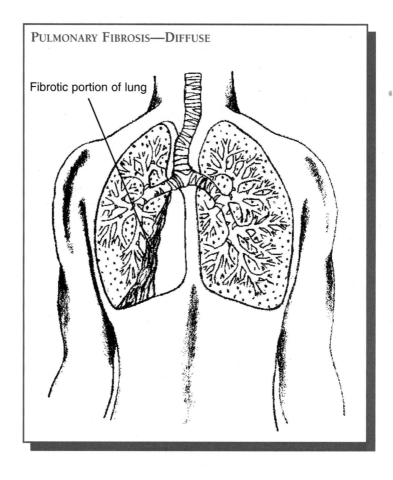

Fibrotic portion of lung

PATHOPHYSIOLOGY

Damage to the lung parenchyma by the inhalation or other exposure to toxic substances results in inflammation or necrosis. As healing occurs, excessive amounts of connective tissue accumulate. As this process continues, structural changes occur in the lungs, with fibrotic tissue gradually replacing the more elastic tissue found normally. Over time, this replacement leads to lung tissue that is stiff and nonelastic. The patient finds it increasingly more difficult to inflate the stiffened lungs. Additionally, the damage may alter gas exchange such that the lungs can no longer meet the body's metabolic demands. Localized fibrosis as a result of infection is generally less severe than diffuse fibrosis.

NURSE ALERT:
Diffuse fibrosis from pneumoconiosis or other toxic exposure is often disabling or fatal.

𝒞hapter 29: Sleep Apnea Syndrome

▽   ▽   ▽   ▽   ▽   ▽   ▽

ℐNTRODUCTION

Periodic cessation of breathing during sleep is called sleep apnea syndrome. It can occur when the airway is obstructed or when activity of respiratory muscles is impaired.

𝒮UPPORTING ASSESSMENT DATA

If your assessment findings are similar to those listed here, they may suggest sleep apnea.

▲ Health History:
- Men over age 50
- Post-menopausal women
- Daytime somnolence
- Snoring
- Headaches, especially in the morning
- Restless movements during sleep
- Personality changes due to loss of sleep
- Decreased libido
- Memory loss or other cognitive impairment

NURSE ALERT:
Patients are generally unaware of breathing patterns during sleep. Bed partners are frequently able to provide the most accurate history.

▲ Physical Findings:
- Hypertension
- Arterial blood gas imbalance
- Enlarged tonsils or uvula
- Excessive tissue in pharynx
- Obesity
- Clinical evidence of hypothyroidism

NURSE ALERT:
While these findings may lead you to suspect sleep apnea, specialized physiologic sleep monitoring can confirm the diagnosis.

PATHOPHYSIOLOGY

Characteristically, two types of breathing patterns lead to sleep apnea. Central apnea is related to impaired neural output with resultant inactivity of respiratory muscles. Obstructive apnea is a result of obstruction of the upper airway.

A mixture of obstructive and central sleep apnea, called mixed apnea, is the most common form of the condition. A combination of factors is involved in the cycle of sleep apnea.

In narrow airways, there is often an increased resistance to airflow and an increased tendency for the airway to collapse. During sleep, the muscles involved in respiration normally operate at reduced levels of activity. Smaller amounts of air enter the lungs, leading to impaired gas exchange.

Eventually, the imbalance becomes so great that the neural controls over respiration trigger increased ventilation. The patient is usually startled out of sleep by this change. Once the patient falls asleep again, the cycle starts over.

SUGGESTED READINGS

Feinsilver, S. H. "Recognizing and Treating the Sleep Apnea Syndromes." *Emergency Medicine* 24, no. 6 (1992): 83–87.

Groth, M. L., and A. N. Hurewitz. "Critical Management of Pleural Effusions: Parapneumonic Effusions and Empyemas." *Emergency Medicine* 22, no. 19 (1990): 111–112, 115–116, 118.

Miller, E. "Breathtaking Experience . . . A Patient's Progress With Severe Right-Sided Pleuritic Pain." *Nursing Times* 88, no. 24 (1992): 36–38.

Twomey, C. R. "Chylothorax in the Adult Heart Transplant Patient: A Case Report." *American Journal of Critical Care* 3, no. 4 (1994): 316–319.

Wilkins, R. L., and J. R. Dexter. "Sleep Apnea in Respiratory Disease." In *Principles of Patient Care.* edited by R. L. Wilkins and J. R. Dexter. Philadelphia: F. A. Davis, 1993.

"When Snoring Signals Danger." *Consumer Reports on Health* 5, no. 12 (1993): 74–78.

INDEX

ORDER OTHER TITLES IN THIS SERIES!

INSTANT NURSING ASSESSMENT:

▲ Cardiovascular	0-8273-7102-0
▲ Respiratory	0-8273-7099-7
▲ Neurologic	0-8273-7103-9
▲ Women's Health	0-8273-7100-4
▲ Gerontologic	0-8273-7101-2
▲ Mental Health	0-8273-7104-7
▲ Pediatric	0-8273-7098-9

RAPID NURSING INTERVENTIONS

▲ Cardiovascular	0-8273-7105-5
▲ Respiratory	0-8273-7095-4
▲ Neurologic	0-8273-7093-8
▲ Women's Health	0-8273-7092-X
▲ Gerontologic	0-8273-7094-6
▲ Mental Health	0-8273-7096-2
▲ Pediatric	0-8273-7097-0

------------------------------ ✂ (cut here) ------------------------------

GET "INSTANT" EXPERIENCE!

QTY.	TITLE / ISBN	PRICE	TOTAL
		19.95	
		19.95	
		19.95	
		19.95	
		19.95	
		19.95	
		SUBTOTAL	
		STATE OR LOCAL TAXES	
		TOTAL	

Payment Information
☐ A Check is Enclosed
☐ Charge my ☐ VISA ☐ Mastercard   CARD #_____

MAIL OR FAX COMPLETED FORM TO:
Delmar Publishers • P.O. Box 15015 • Albany, NY 12212-5015

NAME _____

SCHOOL/INSTITUTION _____

STREET ADDRESS_____

CITY/STATE/ZIP _____

HOME PHONE_____

OFFICE PHONE_____

**IN A HURRY TO ORDER? FAX: 1-518-464-0301
OR CALL TOLL-FREE 1-800-347-7707**